Continuing Education and Lifelong Learning in Social Work

This book focuses on the present development, gradual evolution, and current status of social work continuing education. The contributors demonstrate the rapidly growing importance of continuing education (CE) in the social work profession; look closely at present trends; and address the emerging pedagogical issues that will likely frame the future. The rapid expansion of CE offerings is partly stimulated by CE now being a licensure renewal requirement across the United States, which quite clearly is having a central impact in expanding the demand for CE education and lifelong learning for professional practice.

Relevant for social work students, graduates and educators, in the USA and abroad, this book represents an authoritative statement, authored by widely recognized educators and practitioners who are on the forefront of continuing education and lifelong learning.

This book was originally published as a special issue of the *Journal of Teaching in Social Work*.

Paul A. Kurzman holds a dual appointment as a Professor of Social Work at the Silberman School of Hunter College, USA, and as a Professor of Social Welfare at The Graduate School and University Center of the City University of New York, USA, where he teaches policy and practice in the MSW and PhD programs. He is an author or editor of 10 books, Editor-in-Chief of the *Journal of Teaching in Social Work*, and a frequent provider of continuing education lectures, trainings, and workshops. Dr. Kurzman holds a BA from Princeton University, an MSW from Columbia University, and a PhD from New York University.

Continuing Education and Lifelong Learning in Social Work

Current Issues and Future Direction

Edited by
Paul A. Kurzman

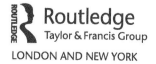

Routledge
Taylor & Francis Group

LONDON AND NEW YORK

First published 2018
by Routledge

2 Park Square, Milton Park, Abingdon, Oxfordshire OX14 4RN
52 Vanderbilt Avenue, New York, NY 10017

Routledge is an imprint of the Taylor & Francis Group, an informa business

First issued in paperback 2019

British Library Cataloguing in Publication Data
A catalogue record for this book is available from the British Library

ISBN 13: 978-1-138-57228-7 (hbk)
ISBN 13: 978-0-367-89253-1 (pbk)

Typeset in Minion
by RefineCatch Limited, Bungay, Suffolk

Publisher's Note
The publisher accepts responsibility for any inconsistencies that may have
arisen during the conversion of this book from journal articles to book chapters,
namely the possible inclusion of journal terminology.

Disclaimer
Every effort has been made to contact copyright holders for their permission to
reprint material in this book. The publishers would be grateful to hear from any
copyright holder who is not here acknowledged and will undertake to rectify
any errors or omissions in future editions of this book.

Contents

CONTENTS

Citation Information

The chapters in this book were originally published in the *Journal of Teaching in Social Work*. When citing this material, please use the original page numbering for each article, as follows:

Chapter 7
The Learning Institute: Promoting Social Justice Advocacy Within a Continuing Education Program
Karen Rice, Heather Girvin, Jennifer Frank, and Leonora Foels
Journal of Teaching in Social Work, volume 36, issue 4 (2016), pp. 380–389

Chapter 8
A Gerontology Practitioner Continuing Education Certificate Program: Lessons Learned
Jacqueline Englehardt, Kristina M. Hash, Mariann Mankowski, Karen V. Harper-Dorton, and Ann E. Pilarte
Journal of Teaching in Social Work, volume 36, issue 4 (2016), pp. 407–420

Chapter 9
Connecting Social Work and Activism in the Arts Through Continuing Professional Education
Kathryn Rawdon and David Moxley
Journal of Teaching in Social Work, volume 36, issue 4 (2016), pp. 431–443

Chapter 10
Creating a Continuing Education Pathway for Newly Arrived Immigrants and Refugee Communities
Aster S. Tecle, An Thi Ha, and Rosemarie Hunter
Journal of Teaching in Social Work, volume 37, issue 2 (2017), pp. 171–184

For any permission-related enquiries please visit:
http://www.tandfonline.com/page/help/permissions

Notes on Contributors

Larry Berkowitz, Ed.D. is Director of the Riverside Trauma Center in Needham, MA, USA.

Joanna Bridger, LICSW is the Clinical Service Director of the Riverside Trauma Center in Needham, MA, USA.

Jacqueline Englehardt, ACSW is Professional and Community Education Director at the School of Social Work of West Virginia University, Morgantown, WV, USA.

Leonora Foels, PhD is an Associate Professor at the School of Social Work of Millersville University, Millersville, PA, USA.

Jennifer Frank, PhD is an Instructor at the School of Social Work of Millersville University, Millersville, PA, USA.

Scott Miyake Geron, PhD is an Associate Professor and Director of the Center for Aging and Disability Education and Research at the School of Social Work of Boston University, Boston, MA, USA.

Mark Gianino, PhD is a Clinical Associate Professor at the School of Social Work of Boston University, Boston, MA, USA.

Heather Girvin, PhD is an Associate Professor and MSW Program Coordinator at the School of Social Work of Millersville University, Millersville, PA, USA.

Charlotte Goodluck, PhD, until her death, was Professor Emerita of Social Work and Sociology at Portland State University, Portland, OR, USA.

An Thi Ha is a PhD candidate at the College of Social Work of the University of Utah, Salt Lake City, UT, USA.

Karen V. Harper-Dorton, PhD is a Professor at the School of Social Work of West Virginia University, Morgantown, WV, USA.

Kristina M. Hash, PhD is a Professor and Gerontology Certificate Director at the School of Social Work of West Virginia University, Morgantown, WV, USA.

Rosemarie Hunter, PhD is an Associate Professor in the College of Social Work at the University of Utah, Salt Lake City, UT, USA.

Pauline Jivanjee, PhD is an Associate Professor at the School of Social Work of Portland State University, Portland, OR, USA.

Paul A. Kurzman, PhD is a Professor of Social Work at the Silberman School of Hunter College, USA, and a Professor of Social Welfare at The Graduate Center of the City University of New York, New York, NY, USA.

Ching Man Lam, PhD is a Professor and Vice-Chairperson of the Department of Social Work at the Chinese University of Hong Kong, Shatin, HK.

Yan Liang, M.Phil is a Research Assistant at the Chinese University of Hong Kong, Shatin, HK.

Mariann Mankowski, PhD is an Assistant Professor at the School of Social Work of West Virginia University, Morgantown, WV, USA.

James McCauley, LICSW is an Associate Director of the Riverside Trauma Center in Needham, MA, USA.

Rebecca G. Mirick, PhD is an Associate Professor at the School of Social Work of Salem State University, Salem, MA, USA.

David Moxley, PhD is a Professor at the Knee Center of the Zarrow School of Social Work at the University of Oklahoma, Norman, OK, USA.

Laura Nissen, PhD is Dean and Professor at the School of Social Work of Portland State University, Portland, OR, USA.

Kimberly Pendell, PhD is an Associate Professor at the Social Work of Portland State University, Portland, OR, USA.

Ann E. Pilarte, MSW is a Home Hospice Social Worker at Hospice and Community Care, Lancaster, PA, USA.

Kathryn Rawdon, MSW is Advocate Supervisor, CASA of Oklahoma County, Oklahoma City, OK, USA.

Karen Rice, PhD is an Associate Professor and Co-Director of the DSW Program at the School of Social Work of Millersville University, Millersville, PA, USA.

Betty J. Ruth, MSW, MPH is a Clinical Professor at the School of Social Work of Boston University, Boston, MA, USA.

Robert Schachter, DSW is the former Executive Director of the New York City Chapter of the National Association of Social Workers, New York, NY, USA.

Aster S. Tecle, PhD is an Assistant Professor in the College of Social Work at the University of Utah, Salt Lake City, UT, USA.

Miu Chung Yan, PhD is a Professor and the Director of the School of Social Work at the University of British Columbia, Vancouver, BC, Canada.

Acknowledgements

When we issued a Call for Papers for a text on *Social Work Continuing Education* we had not imagined the response we would receive. While we knew this to be a cutting-edge issue, which prompted our interest in taking the initiative, the sheer number of excellent manuscripts we received, many for the journal's special issue and hence the book, certainly did pleasantly surprise us. Our belief that the time had come for a new and authoritative text on the subject had been validated, and we hope the peer-reviewed selection of these 10 superb chapters confirms that conviction to the reader. Representing the ideas of 30 contributing authors, the chapters herein present new information, novel experimentation, fresh conceptualization and creative templates for what represents an important thrust for professional social work education for the present and the future.

As Editor, I am very grateful to the can-do spirit and steady support of Abigail Carson, Managing Editor for Behavioral Science and Social Care, Nicholas Barclay, Editor of Routledge Special Issues as Books, and Rachel Dalton, Production Editor at the Taylor & Francis Group. Their patience and flexibility made a difference. And it is clear that this book would not have been possible without the quiet, steady and focused support of Ruth Flaherty, the Assistant Editor of the *Journal of Teaching in Social Work*, who carried out so many of the tasks of assignment and production with an always skillful and steady hand.

And to the contributors, whose insights and innovations are so articulately expressed here, we give thanks and tribute for their remarkable creativity and perspicacity. In this book, each of them individually, and all of them collectively, have made an indelible professional contribution to the topic of continuing education and lifelong learning in the social work profession.

Paul A. Kurzman
September 2017

Preface

Paul A. Kurzman

The rapid growth of continuing education in social work during the past decade is changing academia and expanding the expectations of education for professional practice. This volume focuses on the early development, gradual evolution and current status of social work continuing professional education. Relevant for social work students, educators and graduates, here and abroad, this book represents an authoritative statement authored by widely recognized educators and practitioners who are on the forefront of continuing education and lifelong learning.

Documenting the current state of the art, this comprehensive text demonstrates the growing importance of lifelong learning in the social work profession. The authors look closely at current trends and address the emerging pedagogical issues that will likely frame the future.

Social Work Continuing Education: Current Issues and Future Direction

Paul A. Kurzman

ABSTRACT

Continuing education is arising as an area of rapid growth and increased attention in the social work profession. Conceptually, the impetus and focus are on the promotion of the principles of lifelong learning and professional replenishment; but pragmatically, the driving force has been the virtually universal requirement of continuing education hours for social work licensure renewal. This chapter lays out the history of continuing social work education and discusses the current and emerging issues herein for the profession.

Introduction

Although the core of social work education involves the preparation of future practitioners through the profession's accredited baccalaureate and master's degree programs, increasing emphasis now is being placed on the centrality of continuing education (CE) as a way of ensuring the presence of lifelong learning. Even though this evolving focus is true for virtually all professions, social work is a relative newcomer in this arena.

The growth of CE in social work has had several antecedents and significant sources of support. As Strom-Gottfried (2008) noted, the early impetus in the practice community derived significantly from the passage of the Title XX Amendments to the Social Security Act in 1974, which for the first time provided funds to cover social service staff in-service training. When this funding declined in the 1980s, such training activities did as well, not to reemerge until well into the 1990s, due primarily then to the impetus provided by the expansion of state social work licensing, and the customary requirement that social work licensees obtain units of CE in order to secure licensure renewal (Davenport & Wodarski, 1989; Strom-Gottfried, 2008). In 1998, the academic community also took note of the emerging importance of CE with the founding of a peer-refereed journal titled *Professional Development: The International Journal of Continuing Social Work Education.*

Defined by Halton, Powell, Jivanjee, and Goodluck (2014) as "an ongoing process of education and development that continues throughout the professional career" (p. 1), CE also is commonly known as "lifelong learning" and "continuing professional education." In this sense, CE generally is conceptualized as an element of what Malcolm Knowles (1998) termed "andragogy," that is, "the art and science of helping adults learn" (p. 61). Using a pedagogy specifically adapted for adult education, lifelong learning has come to be seen as a requisite—not a luxury—in a world in which knowledge generation has become so rapid and profound that no professional today can been seen as adequately informed for practice solely based on a prior graduate degree and early career certification (Lam, Wong, Hui, Lee, & Chan, 2006). Hence, the conclusion that CE is a necessity has gradually become widely accepted by members of the social work profession. "Social workers practice in rapidly changing and complex environments where they encounter challenges that include increasing evidence-based practice requirements, a shifting information landscape, and diminishing workplace resources. ... To address these challenges," Nissen, Pendell, Jivanjee, and Goodluck (2014) opined, "social workers need to engage in lifelong learning" (p. 384).

From a pragmatic perspective, there were several major events that provided the decisive stimulus for greater attention to CE during the past decade. First and foremost, of course, was the final passage of mandatory CE requirements for social work licensure renewal in all 50 states (as well as the District of Columbia, U.S. Virgin Islands, Northern Mariana Islands, and Guam). The three final holdouts (Colorado, Hawaii, and New York) gradually joined the other 47 states, with New York as the last state to implement the mandate, effective January 2015. (It is worth noting that New York's decision to come aboard was especially significant because it has 57,000 licensed social workers, far more than any other state in the nation.) The enactment of the New York requirement created both renewed attention to and a greatly expanded market for CE offerings. The Council on Social Work Education (CSWE) evinced an enhanced interest in CE as well, reflected in part by sponsorship of a CE consortium (known as CENET) to bring together its school-based CE directors. However, CSWE's most important influence on CE emanated from the publication of its new Education Policy and Accreditation Standards in 2015, which placed a more explicit emphasis on competency-based education, underscoring that "an individual social worker's competence is seen as developmental and dynamic, changing over time in relation to continued learning" (CSWE, 2015, pp. 2–3). Competence 1, "Demonstrating Ethical and Professional Behavior," specifically noted that social workers should "recognize the importance of life-long learning and ... of continually updating their skills to ensure they are relevant and effective" (CSWE, 2015, pp. 2–3). Meanwhile, the National Association of Social Workers (NASW) had issued its first formal position on the topic, via the publication of a comprehensive *Standards for Continuing Professional Education*, which emphasized that "a commitment to continuing education is grounded in an ethical principle articulated in the NASW *Code of Ethics*," which specifies that social workers must "develop and enhance their professional expertise" (NASW, 2003, p. 9) and "should critically examine and keep current with emerging knowledge relevant to social work" (NASW, 2008, sec. 4.01b). The Code further states that "social work administrators and supervisors should take reasonable steps to provide or arrange for continuing education and staff development for all staff for whom they are responsible" (NASW, 2008, sec. 3.08). In this spirit, NASW now requires members who hold or seek its professional social work credentials (such as the Diplomate in Clinical Social Work), or advanced practice specialty credentials (such as the Qualified Clinical Social Worker or Certified Advanced Social Work Case Manager) to obtain a minimum of 20–30 hours of related continuing education every two years (NASW Credentialing Center, 2015).

Finally, in 2011 the Association of Social Work Boards (ASWB) Foundation for Research and Consumer Education in Social Work Regulation funded social work scholars at the Boston University School of Social Work to conduct an in-depth study of continuing social work education. Termed "The Missing Link Project" and led by Betty J. Ruth, Mark Gianino, and Scott M. Geron (2014a), ASWB's 119-page *Final Report* included a comprehensive survey on the status of CE in the United States and Canada and culminated in a series both of observations and recommendations. Among its strongest superordinate conclusions was "the urgent need for a national conversation, including a call that all of the profession's organizations make CE the 'issue of the year'" (p. 56). The authors firmly believed that "by starting with a structured cross profession dialogue [one will be able to] identify a variety of methods for deepening an approach to lifelong learning in the social work profession" (Ruth, Gianino, & Geron, 2014b, p. 16). They concluded with the hope that "the broader profession's understanding of CE as a crucial, but overlooked, link to quality improvement, practitioner effectiveness, and consumer protection" will measurably be enhanced by their project's explicit research findings (p. 16).

Current Activity

Continuing professional education today is provided by schools of social work, social agencies, professional associations, postgraduate institutes, and individual entrepreneurs who have incorporated in order to provide CE seminars and workshops. In many states, chapters of the major professional organizations (such as NASW) and accredited social work education entities

(MSW and BSW programs) sponsor the largest share of the CE offerings, yet a number of proprietary firms have sprung up in response to the demand. Given that there presently are more than 490,000 licensed social workers (termed "registered social workers" in Canada) in North America today, one can readily appreciate the enticing new market, as virtually all of them will need to obtain CE hours (credits) every year to obtain their periodic state licensure renewal. Some of the present for-profit providers are new entrants into the CE marketplace, such as SocialWorkTodayCE.com, whereas others have been in business for many years—like Coursera, Udacity, and the University of Phoenix. Hence, a new industry has emerged. Some of the proprietary universities and educational corporations seem to be providing CE options of good quality; however, this new entrepreneurial opportunity also has spawned a number of "certificate mills," of dubious merit, that would appear to be primarily focused on shareholder Return on Investment. Because individual state (or territorial) licensing boards make the final determination on what courses, provided by which sponsors, will qualify toward the state-mandated CE credits, there is an opportunity to screen out offerings on inappropriate topics, provided by insufficiently qualified instructors, or presented under unsuitable auspices. Yet, with due respect for the spirit of free enterprise, it is gradually becoming recognized that there may well be inherent risks built in when profit-focused sponsors enter the educational arena (Kurzman, 2015).

The emergence of distance learning and online education has revolutionized education and practice, and the profession of social work has not been an exception. We currently have peer-reviewed electronic journals, and respected BSW, MSW, and DSW degree programs, offered entirely online. Whatever may be the systemic limitations and risks, the online option provides easy access to CE for rural providers, full-time practitioners (balancing work with child and/or elder care), those with physical limitations and disabilities, and multitasking practitioners who prefer the flexibility inherent in home- or office-based course instruction (Noble & Russell, 2013). In short, online options offer intriguing opportunities for broadening and extending access to CE. As we have suggested elsewhere,

> With the advent of broadband availability, more powerful processors, secure interactive video transmission, simulcast broadcasting with ITV, versatile web conferencing software, high-end graphics, avatar assisted animation, and sophisticated web-based platforms, the options for online education (and therefore distance learning) are extensive. (Kurzman, 2013, pp. 332–333)

As the overarching association representing the jurisdictional boards that regulate social work in the United States and Canada, the ASWB membership includes all 50 U.S. states, all 10 Canadian provinces, the District of Columbia, the U.S. Virgin Islands, the U.S. Territory of Guam, and the U.S.

Commonwealth of Northern Mariana Islands (ASWB Guide, 2015a, p. 5). In performing its central function, the ASWB develops and maintains the social work licensing exams (bachelor's, master's, advanced generalist, and clinical) that these jurisdictions may select and deploy. Recognizing that CE (like doctoral social work education) is neither overseen by NASW nor accredited by CSWE, ASWB created an Approved Continuing Education (ACE) program in 2001 to help standardize social work CE approval and identify CE programs that met a set of established criteria. Although NASW's *Standards for Continuing Professional Education* (2003) and *Continuing Education Program Guidelines* (2011) represent authoritative statements, and present a useful paradigm for providers and practitioners, the ASWB's ACE program has established uniform requirements that have proven to be broadly acceptable to social work regulatory boards in many jurisdictions throughout the United States and Canada. In effect, ACE was formed in large part to be able to serve the important function, metaphorically, of providing a Good Housekeeping "seal of approval" in the arena of continuing social work education. In its brochure, ACE sponsors state, "Several national organizations, including ASWB, review CE providers for program quality. Providers who pass these screenings meet stringent requirements for program development and management" (ASWB, n.d.). (For example, approved offerings must be for at least 1 hour, with clearly defined learning objectives, ending with an evaluation measure. Session formats focused on oral presentations, discussion groups, and poster presentations would not meet ACE requirements.) Presently, 47 regulatory jurisdictions accept ACE-approved CE hours (39 U.S. states, six Canadian provinces, the U.S. Virgin Islands, and the District of Columbia). Although New York, with its record 57,000 licensed social workers, is not among the jurisdictions that automatically accept the ACE-screened CE offerings, ASWB today can appropriately claim that "the ACE approved brand is recognized widely as the gold standard for social work CE" (ASWB News, 2015b, p. 2).

Current Issues

Many differences exist among the states and territories with regard to their respective CE requirements. For example, although NASW (2003) specifies that social workers should "complete 48 hours of continuing professional education every 2 years" (p. 12), some jurisdictions mandate more and many require less; some states will accept only CE credits awarded by its own list of preapproved providers; others specify that a certain portion of CE credits must be earned in specific areas such as ethics, cultural competence, substance abuse, HIV-AIDS, or domestic violence prevention. Given that the CE requirement today mainly derives from jurisdictional mandates for licensure renewal, and that all matters pertaining to professional licensing reside with the individual states and territories, one cannot expect uniformity. Moreover, although it is the current practice among virtually all the professions, tying CE almost exclusively to licensure and related credential renewal requirements may well not be an optimal strategy, or learning framework.

As several scholars have remarked, there currently are new, completely independent, and often very legitimate pressures for the social work profession to demonstrate currency and competency in mastering evolving knowledge. We are rightly expected to be deploying empirically supported interventions that constitute evidence-based practice, leading to what we commonly term "best practices" (Kirk & Reid, 2002; Parrish & Rubin, 2011). Consequently, separate from licensure requirements, there is a recognized need to assess CE outcomes in order to validate the impact and effectiveness of professional education. Such is the expectation in accredited BSW and MSW programs, and should be in our postdegree offerings as well. An entirely fair critique of the requisite lectures, workshops, and seminars (which currently can be counted as approved CE hours) is that generally only attendance is assessed and required. (Experientially, as well, we know that such criticism may be justified, as many who have served as CE instructors have commented on the significant number of attendees who, during the sessions, appear to be retrieving their e-mail, sending texts, scanning social media, listening to music, or engaged in playing solitaire.) As a national authority on social work CE has written, "There is little evidence to show that attending myriad continuing education conferences, seminars, classes and online offerings has any correlation to maintaining or improving the skills of a practicing professional" (Hymans, 2007, p. 8).

In this regard, there is support from our sister professions. In an attempt to ascertain the impact of mandated CE, the National Council of State Boards of Nursing conducted a survey of six professions, and their study came forward with two significant findings: The respondents gave CE "relatively minimal credit for their professional development" and "the same amount of professional growth was generally reported by those required by law to have CE, and by those who had no requirement" (ASWB, 2003, p. 15). Further, a pair of studies published in 2015 by the American Medical Association found no correlation whatsoever between mandated physician maintenance of specialty certification CE and better patient outcomes (Kirsch, 2015, p. D-3).

Although social work research has been slim in the area of outcome assessment, a summative study of 230 licensed social workers in Maryland by Charles Smith et al. (2006) found that self-perceived change scores were significantly higher for informal versus formal CE. The study authors also observed that there is a dearth of evidence to support the case that social workers' CE participation does, in fact, improve practice. Hence, merely fulfilling CE requirements, as a variable, may indeed increase knowledge but does not appear to necessarily improve competency, and thereby enhance professional practice. Moreover, these findings would seem to be supported by the research observations of professional colleagues (Cochran & Landuyt, 2010; Mansouri & Lockyer, 2007).

The pivotal issues of impact and outcome assessment have been well stated by Elaine Congress (2012), who noted, "Although there has been much focus on evidence-based practice, the evaluation of the effectiveness of continuing education programs has been minimal" (p. 400). Most postprogram evaluations continue to rely on an assessment of attendees' levels of satisfaction, along with a request for participants' perceptions of knowledge gained—and both are weak measures, at best. In fact, little effort has been made to conduct longitudinal evaluations to ascertain, for example, whether the new knowledge is retained or is merely temporal in nature. Even more important, little energy to date has been devoted by CE providers to discovering whether the knowledge transmitted has been converted into new competencies that have moved program participants toward evidence-based "best practices" in their service sector. In sum, there would appear to be a serious shortage of research directed toward proof of the effectiveness of the ever-growing number of social work CE options.

Conclusion and Additional Issues

Given that CE is widely mandated today in the social work profession, and therefore the more than 490,000 licensed social workers in North America are actively pursuing CE study each year, a more rigorous measurement of program outcomes must be conceptualized and implemented. Because all education for entry into the social work profession, via our CSWE-accredited BSW and MSW programs, is expected to follow the principles of competency-based education (CSWE, 2015), the profession and its agents have an obligation as well to institute formative and summative competency-focused assessments of postdegree lifelong learning initiatives embodied in their CE offerings. CE is like doctoral social work education (Kurzman, 2015); both are still largely unregulated arenas that do not require curricular approval from a national professional organization or accreditation by a nationally recognized body. Thus, whatever discipline and rigor will be infused in the future in this field of endeavor will likely have to be at the initiative of leaders and scholars of the profession.

Although the thoughtful authors of the chapters share their views, experiences, findings, and insights, we would underscore that the discussion presented here merely represents a historical and conceptual framework for the principal prevailing issues in the sphere of continuing professional education. The collective strengths and limitations, challenges and achievements, struggles and accomplishments, are far too numerous to list. This reality, of course, is true for most educational programs in this complex and ever-changing world. We would nonetheless be remiss at this juncture if we were not to make brief mention of several other questions and quandaries facing social work CE today. In our judgment they too are worthy of wide discussion and debate. They would include the following:

- What would represent the optimal CE pedagogy for social work in the United States?
- Does current social work CE achieve the goal of enhancing, advancing, and enriching social work practice?
- Do social work CE offerings currently meet the unique needs of macro social work practitioners?
- What are the appropriate roles of CSWE, NASW, and ASWB in establishing national CE standards for the social work profession?
- Given the central role of accessibility, to what degree should home-based study, online programs, CD-ROM and Webinar options (and similar self-paced instructional formats) be promoted as pathways for completing CE units of study?
- What can the United States learn about effective CE from its present practice in other countries?
- Should CE become competency based, rather than focused primarily on participation and hours of attendance?
- What organizations are likely to be the most appropriate providers of social work CE: major professional associations, accredited social work education programs, proprietary CE providers, recognized postgraduate institutes, or public and nonprofit social agencies?
- Should the cost of obtaining requisite CE units be borne solely by practitioners, or be shared by agencies and employers?
- To what degree do the current NASW Standards for Continuing Professional Education represent an appropriate template for the social work profession?
- Should the Group for the Advancement of Doctoral Education promote the topic of CE as an area for doctoral dissertation inquiry?
- Do current social work CE providers adequately measure the learning outcomes of their participants?
- As there is national accreditation for baccalaureate and master's degree programs, should there be similar universal accreditation for social work CE programs?
- To what extent is CE a staff development responsibility of social work employers?
- How can CE providers ensure that their offerings are continuously responsive to the expectations and evolving needs of those enrolled?
- Is CE the optimal way to promote and ensure lifelong professional learning?

This text, in part, is responsive to ASWB's seminal study of CE in social work (titled the Missing Link Project, and noted earlier), which strongly recommended that key stakeholders concerned with the quality of social work practice "begin a national conversation about the state of CE in social work" and specifically encourage "one or more major social work journals to dedicate an issue or supplement to CE issues" (Ruth et al., 2014a, p. 57). Here we have sought to solicit the advice of some of the wisest scholars committed to the enhancement of CE for our profession. It is our hope that, collectively, the authors here will be able to make a modest contribution to offering remedies that will prove as comprehensive as the need.

References

Association of Social Work Boards. (2003). Research: Mandated CE may not be as effective as thought. *ASWB Association News, 13*(3), 15–16.

Association of Social Work Boards. (2015a). *ASWB guide to the social work exams.* Culpeper, VA: Author.

Association of Social Work Boards. (2015b). Your board in action. *ASWB Association News, 25*(4), 2.

Association of Social Work Boards. (n.d.). *Continuing education: A guide for social workers.* Culpeper, VA: Author.

Cochran, G., & Landuyt, N. (2010). A survey of continuing education programs conducted. *Professional Development: The International Journal of Continuing Social Work Education, 13*(2), 55–72.

Congress, E. P. (2012). Guest editorial, Continuing Education: Lifelong learning for social work practitioners and educators. *Journal of Social Work Education, 48*(3), 397–401. doi:10.5175/JSWE.2012.201200085

Council on Social Work Education. (2015). *Final 2015 educational policy statement.* Alexandria, VA: Author.

Davenport, J., & Wodarski, J. S. (1989). Social work continuing education: An historical description. *Arete, 14*, 32–45.

Final report: The Missing Link Project. (2014, November/December). *ASWB Association News, 24*(6), 1–2.

Halton, C., Powell, F., Jivanjee, P., & Goodluck, C. (2014). *Continuing professional development in social work.* London, UK: Policy Press.

Hymans, D. (2007, December). Conference ponders if there is a better way to ensure continued competency. *ASWB Association News,* p. 8, 13.

Kirk, S. A., & Reid, W. J. (2002). *Science and social work: A critical appraisal.* New York, NY: Columbia University Press.

Knowles, M. (1998). *The adult learner.* Houston, TX: Gulf Publishing.

Krisch, J. A. (2015, April 14). A voluntary test in name only. *The New York Times,* p. D3.

Kurzman, P. A. (2013). The evolution of distance learning and online education. *Journal of Teaching in Social Work, 33*, 331–338. doi:10.1080/08841233.2013.843346

Kurzman, P. A. (2015). The evolution of doctoral social work education. *Journal of Teaching in Social Work, 35*, 1–13. doi:10.1080/08841233.2015.1007832

Lam, D. O. B., Wong, D. K. P., Hui, S. H. K., Lee, F. W. L., & Chan, E. K. L. (2006). Preparing social workers to be lifelong learners. *Journal of Teaching in Social Work, 26*, 103–119. doi:10.1300/J067v26n03_07

Mansouri, M., & Lockyer, J. (2007). A meta-analysis of continuing medical education effectiveness. *Journal of Continuing Education in the Health Professions, 27*(1), 6–15. doi:10.1002/chp.88

National Association of Social Workers. (2003). *Standards for continuing professional education*. Washington, DC: NASW Press.

National Association of Social Workers. (2008). *Code of ethics*. Washington, DC: NASW Press.

National Association of Social Workers. (2011). *Continuing education program guidelines*. Washington, DC: NASW Press.

National Association of Social Workers Credentialing Center. (2015). *NASW Professional Social Work Credentials and Advanced Specialty Practice Credentials*. Retrieved from http://www.naswdc.org/credentials/list.asp

Nissen, L., Pendell, K., Jivanjee, P., & Goodluck, C. (2014). Lifelong learning in social work education: A review of the literature and implications for the future. *Journal of Teaching in Social Work, 34*(4), 384–400. doi:10.1080/08841233.2014.936577

Noble, D., & Russell, A. C. (2013). Research on webbed connectivity in a web-based learning environment: Online social work education. *Journal of Teaching in Social Work, 33*, 496–513. doi:10.1080/08841233.2013.829167

Parrish, D. E., & Rubin, A. (2011). An effective model for continuing education training in evidence-based practice. *Research on Social Work Practice, 21*(1), 77–87. doi:10.1177/1049731509359187

Ruth, B. J., Gianino, M., & Geron, S. M. (2014a). *The ASWB missing link project final report*. Retrieved from http://www.aswb.org/wp.../11/missing-link-final-report-10_9-final.pdf

Ruth, B. J., Gianino, M., & Geron, S. M. (2014b). *The ASWB missing link project executive summary*. Boston, MA: Boston University School of Social Work.

Smith, C. A., Cohen-Callow, A., Dia, D. A., Bliss, D. L., Gantt, A., Cornelius, L. J., & Harrington, D. (2006). Staying current in a changing profession: Evaluating perceived change resulting from continuing professional education. *Journal of Social Work Education, 42*, 465–482. doi:10.5175/JSWE.2006.042310002

Strom-Gottfried, K. (2008). Continuing education. In T. Mizrahi & L. E. Davis (Eds.), *Encyclopedia of social work* (20th ed., Vol. 1, pp. 451–453). Washington, DC: NASW Press.

Lifelong Learning in Social Work Education: A Review of the Literature and Implications for the Future

LAURA NISSEN

KIMBERLY PENDELL

PAULINE JIVANJEE, and CHARLOTTE GOODLUCK

Social workers practice in rapidly changing and complex environments where they encounter challenges that include increasing evidence-based practice requirements, a shifting information landscape, and diminishing workplace resources. To address these challenges, social workers need to engage in lifelong learning. The purpose of this article is to explore conceptual elements and assumptions underlying lifelong learning; propose social work specific approaches to lifelong learning; present a conceptual model to orient social work educators to the possibilities inherent in lifelong learning for practice, with inclusion of suggested practice behavior; and offer a research agenda for practice.

INTRODUCTION

People who work in professions such as social work, medicine, and education are experiencing turbulence, change, and increasing complexity at unprecedented levels. Many assert that the very nature of most professional work has shifted to a "knowledge economy," defined by Powell and Snellman (2004) as one that balances "production and services, based on knowledge-intensive activities that contribute to an accelerated pace of technical and scientific advance as well as rapid obsolescence" (p. 199). To survive in this new economy, some say that our collective focus must shift toward becoming a "learning society" (Morgan-Klein & Osborne, 2007; Wain, 2000; Walters, 2010). Professional preparation programs acknowledge that professional identity is best grounded in an understanding that knowledge needs to be renewed, expanded, challenged, and redefined throughout a given career (Gardiner & Kline, 2007; Kasworm & Hemminsen, 2007; Kirby, Knapper, Lamon, & Eganoff, 2010; Lewis, 1998). Professionals are being scrutinized with increased rigor due to the growing demands of interest groups, stakeholders, and consumers. In this contemporary context, Deakin-Crick and Wilson (2005) described lifelong learning as "an essential life skill" (p. 359), and both formal and informal learning are becoming key elements of a life well lived, success in the new economy, and a healthy society.

Social work finds itself at the intersection of innovation, expanding knowledge, and external scrutiny. Although ours is a profession with a recognized body of knowledge (Bartlett, 2003; Hare, 2004; Holosko, 2003; Staniforth, Fouché, & O'Brien, 2011), this knowledge is in a continual state of evolution, critique, and development (Carey & Foster, 2011; Feit, 2003; Leslie & Cassano, 2003; Risler, Lowe, & Nackerud, 2003). An example of the changing foundation of social work knowledge is a rapidly emerging set of evidence-based practices to address issues and social problems (Barth et al., 2012; Proctor, 2007; Walker, Briggs, Koroloff, & Friesen, 2007), though such practices have become controversial in their development and design when applied to diverse populations (Bernal & Scharron-Del-Rio, 2001; McBeath, Briggs, & Aisenberg, 2010), depending on the degree to which these client populations have had a role in developing definitions of the problem and successful resolutions (Cross et al., 2011). Reflecting a British perspective, one author warns that social work is subtly shifting from work that focuses on relationships and deep understanding of both situations and context to a profession that collects, manages, and activates transactions based on more superficial information (Parton, 2008). Other authors describe how continuing pressure to attend to marketplace concerns is eroding the value base of the social work profession by conforming to economic pressures (Aronson & Smith, 2011; Reisch, 2011; Schram & Silverman, 2011).

In addition to these shifts, social work education is changing from a knowledge-based curriculum structure to a competency-based one, introducing a myriad of new conceptual and pedagogical factors (Council on Social Work Education [CSWE], 2008; Petracchi & Zastrow, 2010a, 2010b). Competency-based education often is framed as a reaction to the contemporary call for accountability from the public who want to be assured that professionals can demonstrate more than an ability to know something well but that they also can translate that knowledge into effective practice (Hackett, 2001). However, competency-based education is not without its critics, some of whom claim that it is part of a larger effort to restrict, regulate, and control knowledge (Jones & Moore, 1993). As part of the shift to a competency-based paradigm, social work educators are being asked to assure that their graduates can demonstrate skills associated with being a "career-long learner" (CSWE, 2008) and that they will begin their careers fully embracing the imperative to renew and update, as well as challenge, their knowledge and skills continually. The terms "continuing professional education," "career-long learning" and "lifelong learning" often are used interchangeably in adult education settings and discourses. Because we were interested more in the aspirational and ongoing evolution of professionals and their identities (rather than mere compliance with external continuing education requirements), the authors chose to embrace the terminology "lifelong learning" for their review and analysis, finding it fit better with their interest in the lifelong and integrative learning "life" of a professional practitioner.

The concept of lifelong learning relates to a set of values and principles regarding the role of ongoing acquisition, integration, and application of new knowledge throughout one's lifetime, and also includes the practices and structures that position professionals to be relevant, effective, and engaged in their career. Nevertheless, it is both a complex and contested term. Embedded within the lifelong learning literature, a conflict is apparent between multiple ideologies related to the location, purpose, and drivers of learning as both a process and an outcome (Coffield, 1999; Frost, 2001; Jarvis, 2006; Olssen, 2006).

Although a robust literature exists regarding lifelong education in the professions (Frost, 2001; Gustavsson, 2002; Lewis, 1998; Morgan-Klein & Osborne, 2007; Wain, 2000), there is only preliminary coverage of the topic in social work scholarship literature (Congress, 2012; Cournoyer & Stanley, 2002; Daley, 2001; Parrish & Rubin, 2011; Smith et al., 2006). This paucity of inclusion underscores an urgent issue, given the new requirements by the CSWE to embed explicit preparation in this area in social work curricula.

The purpose of this article is multifold. First, it seeks to explore the conceptual elements and assumptions of lifelong learning, propose social work specific approaches to lifelong learning that inform practice behaviors for inclusion in social work education, suggest an evolving practice framework to guide social work education in future years, and offer a research agenda. The authors suggest that to promote, enhance, and embed an orientation toward lifelong learning into social work education and practice, educators be *deliberate and intentional* about building updated lifelong learning models into *social work practice frameworks and educational structures*.

DEFINING LIFELONG LEARNING

For the most part, definitions of lifelong learning focus on the learner and the process and characteristics of learning that normally occur throughout a lifespan. The characteristics of lifelong learning, as outlined by Lewis (1998, p. 62), are that it

- be lifelong (from the cradle to the grave),
- lead to the systematic increase of a person's knowledge and skills, and result in an attitudinal change,
- promote self-fulfillment (professional development) as its ultimate goal,
- strive to increase the learner's ability to be self-directed in learning, and
- acknowledge the contribution of all available educational influences (the learning society).

However, most authors on the subject of lifelong learning agree that simple definitions veil both complexity and conflict. Such complexity refers to the context, influences, opportunities, power differentials, and learner characteristics that may encourage or inhibit such lifelong learning.

To further contextualize and advance a definition of lifelong learning in social work, a few definitions are utilized to form the foundation for the additional proposals presented in this article. The theories reviewed include those that are more functionalist in orientation and focus on continuing education in the service of a career or system, as well as those that reflect some degree of conflict. Conflict theory acknowledges power differentials and context, centering the continually developing person (in this case, the social worker) within complex and often conflict-laden community and organizational settings. Each category represents a subset of the expansive scholarship available on the topic of lifelong learning:

1. Lifelong learning is distinct from, though related to, lifelong education.
2. Lifelong learning relates to professional maintenance, and thus introduces tensions between democratic ideals and economic drivers.
3. Lifelong learning is about personal and professional evolution.
4. Lifelong learning relates to the need for learning organizations.

Lifelong Learning Is Distinct from, Though Related to, Lifelong Education

Billet (2010) drew what he considers to be important distinctions between lifelong learning and lifelong education. By his definition, lifelong learning is both a social process and an intimate and uniquely individual experience, whereas lifelong education (sometimes referred to as continuing education) is an institutional framework for understanding one way of delivering information to adult learners. Further, lifelong learning is a natural and necessary process, and a combination of both individual and group experiences usually aimed at problem solving. Billet stated that lifelong learning is a larger construct than merely being contained or governed by any organizations; rather, it is "essential not only to ourselves and those close to us, but also to the remaking and transformation of the society in which we live" (p. 403). This framework helps social workers recognize and respect that meaningful lifelong learning is not something separate from their personal lives, the lives of the people they work with, or their communities, and that not all continuing learning may come from conferences, books, or trainings.

Lifelong Learning Relates to Professional Maintenance and Introduces Tensions Between Democratic Ideals and Economic Drivers

Frost (2001) described a crisis among professional ranks that relates directly to the speed of change in knowledge and technology, combined with growing diversity, that render any body of knowledge vulnerable from a postmodern standpoint. Legitimacy is being tested in unprecedented ways given that diverse societies "no longer have a shared value base and diverse social groups can challenge their claims to 'objective' knowledge and expertise" (p. 10). Combining a "recognition of social change, the challenge of working with diversity, and the need to constantly renew knowledge claims" (p. 12), Frost asserted the importance of a professional commitment to lifelong learning that may trouble existing canons of knowledge and the need to ensure that reflective professional attitudes and skills incorporate a "recognition of vulnerability to one's own claims to expertise" (p. 14). This framework reinforces the need for social workers to continually explore the foundations of their profession for evidence of both effectiveness and continued adherence to professional values.

Gustavsson (2002) observed that the current generation has witnessed an erosion of concepts associated with the democratic ideals of lifelong learning for the common good. Instead, the evolving language attempts to frame lifelong learning primarily as part of an "economic vocabulary," including gradual deemphasis of the "humanistic concepts with social implications to being defined as human capital" (p. 14). Olssen (2006) noted that society is entering a period of "knowledge capitalism" in which knowledge itself, and control of it through marketplace drivers, is increasingly the norm. Furthermore, the "competency movement" is cited as evidence of this dynamic, along with the dangers associated with its reductionist demands, collapsing complex human interactions into mechanistic acts and economic units (Walters, 2012, p. 201). This discussion of lifelong learning is important because it introduces a larger sociopolitical context including, but not limited to, power analysis and dynamics in play.

Lifelong Learning Is About Personal and Professional Evolution

Based on the early work of Schoen (1982, 1987), Lester (1995) suggested that professions are rapidly evolving past the developmental stages in which the focus was on "applying a body of expert knowledge to known situations in order to produce rational solutions to problems" (p. 44). Contemporary professionals need to "construct and reconstruct the knowledge and skill they need and continually evolve their practice," including the ability to incorporate skills such as "reflecting, inquiring, and creating, which underpin both creative professional practice and academically rigorous learning" (Lester, 1995, p. 44). This body of knowledge is primarily considered to be focused on integrative learning, which Knowles (1990) expressed as a focus on self-directed discovery, knowledge, and integration. Peet and colleagues (2011) described a conceptual framework including elements such as the ability to understand and adapt knowledge gained from a number of sources, experiment reflectively in a variety of situations in order to create positive solutions, organize one's own plan of learning based on emergent needs, and seek feedback from others about one's practice. For professional social workers, this structure is valuable because it centers on adult human development throughout the life span and assumes a positive evolution that will increase humility, effectiveness, and life satisfaction.

Walters (2012) asserted that continual learning by professionals to deal with real-world challenges mandates something deeper than simply "new information, skills or tools." It requires new ways of professional navigation of environments that are rife with "the complex interplay of individual behavior, politics, culture, economics, gender relations, power, and history" in ways that "weave through our personal, political and pedagogical lives" (p. 195). Professionals ideally respond to the resulting ethical dilemmas and human struggle in ways that bring about change and reconciliation through cultivation of a deep respect for the "cultural, spiritual and intimate aspects of peoples' lives" (Walters, 2012, p. 197). Such form of engagement requires learning, skill development, and demonstration, challenging professionals to recognize the complexities and intersectionalities present in professional problem solving as well as their limitations in creating solutions to them.

Lifelong Learning Relates to the Need for Learning Organizations

Frost (2001) stressed that a focus on individual lifelong learning can only take one so far—at some point, lifelong learning advocates must turn their attention to organizational contexts that either promote or inhibit organizational learning. This concept was introduced into the mainstream literature by Senge (1990), who defined the learning organization as one that promotes creativity, problem solving at multiple levels, and development of reflective stances among all members of organizations to read both successes and failures as opportunities to improve, grow, and learn. Cheetham and Chivers (2001) studied how professionals learn in the process of doing their work, identifying a variety of learning mechanisms that helped them become "fully competent professionals, this point often not having been reached until long after their formal professional training had ended" (p. 248). The identified mechanisms are as follows:

1. Practice and repetition
2. Reflection
3. Observation and copying
4. Feedback
5. Extra-occupational transfer
6. Stretching activities
7. Perspective changing/switching
8. Mentor/coach interaction
9. Unconscious absorption or osmosis
10. Use of psychological devices/tricks
11. Articulation
12. Collaboration

This paradigm is important because, although a focus on individual abilities, behaviors, and attitudes is relevant, impact would likely be achieved only as long as there was a simultaneous commitment to organizational development, and the cultivation of organizational leaders who value learning organizations, and know how to construct and maintain them. Numerous examples of this framework have been investigated in practice (Brown & Duguid, 1991; Goldman, 2009; Yang, Watkins, & Marsick, 2004; Yeo, 2005).

Having just explored the various broader conceptualizations of lifelong learning, the focus of this article now shifts to lifelong learning specifically in social work.

LOCATING LIFELONG LEARNING IN SOCIAL WORK

To assure careful positioning of this topic in social work and social work education, some review of our professional grounding may be helpful. According to Gambrill (2006), social workers have three major functions: relief of psychological distress and material need, social control, and social reform (p. 5). These functions translate into services designed to bring about change in some way by providing individual, family, or group therapy, counseling, or support, or by collaborating with others to guide or support organizational or community change. The National Association of Social Workers (2012) reported that nearly 600,000 people have accredited degrees in social work, and according to the Bureau of Labor Statistics (2012), the need for professional social workers is expected to continue to grow by 25% between 2010 and 2020. Demand for social workers is expected to grow even faster in some fields of practice such health care (34%) and mental health and substance abuse (31%; Bureau of Labor Statistics, 2012).

The rapid change and unpredictability in today's environment have resulted in social workers (and other professionals) needing "to be independent, self-directed, autonomous learners" (Taylor, 1997, p. 5). Social workers need to be able to practice with clients of social work services and work collaboratively with members of other professions. Competence, critical self-assessment, and feedback both from peers and consumers are critical in shaping the developing professional (Taylor, 1997).

Social workers are expected to engage in continuing education for their professional development, sometimes arranged or approved by the National Association of Social Workers, and usually as a requirement of maintaining professional licensure in their state. In addition, educational supervision is geared to teaching social workers what they need to know to provide services to the specific types of clients served by their agency (Kadushin & Harkness, 2002). Many agencies provide in-service training for staff as well as case-focused consultation, training, and mentoring by senior staff.

The emphasis on evidence-based practice in social work over the past decade has privileged findings from rigorous research studies, particularly randomized controlled trials, and has required social workers to pursue lifelong learning to be able to deliver interventions with the most substantial research support (Gibbs & Gambrill, 2002). (Critics of the evidence-based practice approach also favor lifelong learning, but for other reasons.) Communities of color, however, frequently have questioned the relevance of traditional social work education for meeting their community-defined needs and have often advocated for social workers' need to learn from community members if they propose to provide culturally responsive services, supported by indigenous ways of knowing (Cross et al., 2011; Huang, Hepburn, & Espiritu, 2003; Isaacs, Huang, Hernandez, & Echo-Hawk, 2005; Lowery, 1998). The concept of professional expertise has been questioned as well by consumer advocacy groups, such as the National Federation of Families for Children's Mental Health and the National Alliance for Mental Illness, which propose more collaborative forms of social work practice, with social workers and clients learning continuously from each other (Slaton, 2003).

Many articles in the social work literature examine the current development of social work's professional identity (Barrett, 2004; Butler, Ford, & Tregaskis, 2007; Hawkins, Fook, & Ryan, 2001; Randall & Kindiak, 2008; Zeira & Rosen, 2000), but there is far less coverage of how social workers incorporate new information as they move through their careers. Surprisingly, the authors were able to locate only a small number of contemporary articles that specifically explored some aspect of the idea of lifelong learning, or its less conceptually robust relation, continuing education. Parish and Rubin

(2011) conducted an exploratory study to examine if training had an impact on understanding and incorporation of evidence-based practices and found that training did have a positive effect. Smith and colleagues (2006) explored how both formal and informal continuing professional education impacted "participants' self-perceived change in knowledge, attitudes and behavior" (p. 465).

Lam, Wong, Hui, Lee, and Chan (2006) devised a study in which use of problem-based learning was utilized to boost students' ownership of social work problem solving in order to increase their "repertoire of learning skills" (p. 112) specifically related to self-directed learning. These skills included "identifying one's own learning needs, conducting one's own exploration of knowledge, evaluating and applying learned material to solve problems, and freedom in deciding what one was going to learn" (p. 112). Although the findings were unclear regarding whether the approach resulted in actual lifelong learning, the authors perceived that it added to the probability that lifelong learning would occur.

Perhaps the most robust of the studies was by Daley (2001), who compared learning by social work professionals with learning by law, adult education, and nursing professionals in order to assert that learning occurs most meaningfully when learners move iteratively between their learning and their professional roles. Social workers specifically identified that the degree to which they could use continuing education to advocate for clients and to create inspiration in their work acted as a reminder "of why they had chosen social work in the first place" (p. 44). All of the professionals in this study described some kind of process that was essential to the type of learning that was most valued by them:

> Professionals described how . . . new information learned in [continuing professional education] programs was added to a professional's knowledge through a complex process of thinking about, acting on, and identifying their feelings about new information. . . . Transferring information to practice was essential to the process of meaning making because often, in this process of using information, the professionals again changed what the information meant to them based on the results they observed. In other words, incorporating new knowledge is a recursive, transforming processing, rather than a simple, straightforward transfer of information from one context to another. (Daley, 2001, p. 50)

Finally, Cournoyer and Stanley (2002) offered a preliminary definition of lifelong learning in social work, the only example of a social work specific definition that could be identified:

> Lifelong learning for social work refers to ongoing processes associated with the acquisition or construction of information, knowledge, and

understanding; the development, adoption, and reconsideration of values and attitudes; and the development of skills and expertise through coursework, experience, observation, conversation, and study from the time someone first explores social work as an educational or professional career choice to the time that person no longer considers him- or herself as a social worker. Lifelong learning experiences can be formal (e.g. a college course or professional seminar) or informal (e.g., an enlightening conversation with another person or a tragic but meaningful life experience). They may be self-initiated or guided by others, independent or collaborative and planned or unplanned. (p. 4)

Based on this definition, the authors also developed an instrument to measure lifelong learning among social workers. As part of an overall framework to encourage the use of social work learning portfolios, Cournoyer and Stanley's instrument includes items such as regular review of professional literature, enjoyment of learning, systematic pursuit of learning activities and opportunities, openness to feedback from others, knowledge of one's personal learning style and preferences, active engagement (with and responsibility for) one's own learning plan, and enjoyment of teaching others. However, no information was available indicating that the scale has been utilized in additional research in program development or in schools of social work and practice settings.

EVOLVING THE DEFINITION OF LIFELONG LEARNING IN SOCIAL WORK PRACTICE TOWARD A MODEL

Whereas the Cournoyer and Stanley (2002) definition of lifelong learning in social work is distinctive for attempting to promote ongoing education for practitioners throughout their careers, the field itself has not continued to develop this conceptual framework beyond a welcome, but only preliminary dialogue (Congress, 2012). Given the CSWE's 2008 Educational Policy and Accreditation Standards (EPAS) requirement to produce graduates who are able to engage in career-long learning, there is an urgent need to be more assertive in the application of this definition.

Figure 1 is a preliminary visual representation of an updated practice paradigm of lifelong learning for social work education. This model is designed with social work students in mind and forms a foundation to ground behaviors related to lifelong learning. In the figure, lifelong learning is centered, with the surrounding components being *knowledge, values,* and *skills*.

Knowledge refers to the importance of understanding the accumulated historical perspective on one's chosen field, current and emerging evidence-informed practices, and an understanding of how rapidly change has and

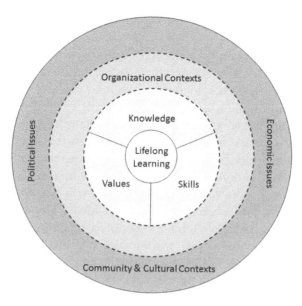

FIGURE 1 Preliminary practice model of lifelong learning for social work education.

will continue to occur. For the purposes of this model, knowledge exists on a continuum ranging from formal to informal, with many gradations in between. Knowledge is dynamic, evolving, and socially constructed. In addition, knowledge includes specific sources of key information of all kinds, necessary to remain relevant and effective in practice.

Values refers to the need for social workers to continually connect lifelong learning to their values and cultivate an understanding that new developments in research and practice should be carefully evaluated through the lens of professional ethics. Also, *values* establishes an ethical obligation for social workers to guide their own plan of lifelong learning, rather than relinquish control of such an important role to a licensing authority or credentialing organization. The idea of merely complying with requirements diminishes the scope, power, and transformational possibilities of professional development, particularly with regard to knowledge and skills that may not be valued by licensing authorities, funders or credentialing organizations.

Skills refers to the ability to develop, refresh, and prioritize a personal plan of lifelong learning, including the ability to seek out new and relevant knowledge for practice. An important aspect of lifelong learning skills is the ability to locate relevant and sound information, both formally in scholarly literature and informally by way of cultivating relationships with consumers and community members.

The next concentric circle represents the *organizational contexts* that social workers can expect to work within. Individual passion for lifelong learning can only go so far if the organizational infrastructure does not support such learning.

Finally, the last concentric circle represents the dynamic *community and cultural context* for social work practice. Preparing students to acknowledge both relevant political issues, including essential skills of conducting power analysis at the community level, including skills related to matters of distributive justice, completes the process of understanding the larger ecological context for their practice and focuses attention on the need to refresh and renew one's practice orientation to these dimensions as well.

Having outlined a conceptual framework for lifelong learning, the next task for social work educators is to robustly evolve a way of articulating a practice behavior that is inclusive of these ideas. The positioning of the career-long learning practice behavior is noted in EPAS Competency 2.1.1: "Identify as a professional social worker and conduct oneself accordingly" (CSWE, 2008). The authors offer the following practice behavior as a beginning of the capacity building process for lifelong learning in social work education:

> Articulate a specific personal/professional plan of lifelong learning which is inclusive of relevant social work knowledge, values, and skills that connect to a commitment to organizational learning (where appropriate) and is reflective of a diverse and dynamic community and cultural context.

The presence of such a practice behavior, alongside the forms of knowledge outlined in this article, lends itself to inclusion of deliberate social work education activities that will ensure that BSW and MSW social work graduates leave their educational experience with a personal, focused, and rigorous framework for lifelong learning. Medicine appears to have particularly well-developed literature on this topic that might be adapted or redefined for the social work profession through introduction of a required "learning for life" module. Such a standard presently lays out a useful conceptual framework to help new physicians envision their lifelong learning needs, methods and intentions (Panda & Desbiens, 2010).

FUTURE RESEARCH

This discourse presents a provocative set of possibilities for the social work profession to consider, debate, and prospectively integrate into how social workers think about pathways to lifelong learning and a related research agenda. Additional research could focus on how definitions of lifelong learning apply in contemporary social work educational and practice settings, the process by which practitioners formally and informally currently create lifelong learning plans, how social workers develop practice questions when faced with work-related challenges, and the manner in which social workers acquire and use ongoing learning as they engage in their work. More information also is needed about the social-work-specific regulatory infrastructure, including how state licensing boards define and operationalize these concepts and mandates.

In the context of the 2008 EPAS, research is needed, as well, regarding the ways that social work education is attempting to meet the challenge of building lifelong-learning-related practice behaviors into student acculturation and professional socialization. This includes the acquisition of information about the instructional methods being used and the degree to which these methods are effective in cultivating graduating social workers who are motivated to continue learning and be connected to a professional lifelong plan. As we move forward with such an agenda, an examination of how other health and mental health professions continue to engage with lifelong learning would be beneficial.

CONCLUSION

Lifelong learning is an important area of emerging social work discourse and presents unique challenges and opportunities to move the social work profession forward. This article has reviewed the lifelong learning literature for social work and beyond and offered preliminary suggestions for ways that social work education and the organized profession might evolve their application and integration of these ideas.

Changing practice, emerging knowledge, and new information sources are abundant; however, time and opportunities to learn and utilize them often are in short supply. As with all matters of the development of social work education's professional trajectory, better that the profession lead the charge to grow its capacity and respond to changes, lest the profession be regulated to do so in ways that may not comport to social work values. This article asserts that there has never been a more relevant time to craft models and structures to advance our capacity to become effective lifelong learners.

REFERENCES

Aronson, J., & Smith, K. (2011). Identity work and critical social service management: Balancing on a tightrope? *British Journal on Social Work, 41,* 432–448.

Barrett, M. (2004). What do we know about the professional socialization of our students? *Journal of Social Work Education, 40,* 255–283.

Barth, R. P., Lee, B. R., Lindsey, M. A., Collins, K. S., Strieder, F., Chorpita, B. F., . . . Sparks, J. A. (2012). Evidence-based practice at a crossroads: The timely emergence of common elements and common factors. *Research on Social Work Practice, 22,* 108–119.

Bartlett, H. M. (2003). Working definition of social work practice. *Research on Social Work Practice, 3,* 5–8.

Bernal, G., & Scharron-Del-Rio, M. R. (2001). Are empirically supported treatments valid for ethnic minorities? Toward an alternative approach for treatment research. *Cultural Diversity and Ethnic Minority Psychology, 7,* 328–342.

Billet, S. (2010). The perils of confusing lifelong learning with lifelong education. *International Journal of Lifelong Education, 29,* 401–413.

Brown, J. S., & Duguid, P. (1991). Organizational learning and communities of practice: Toward a unified view of working, learning, and innovation. *Organizational Science, 2,* 40–57.

Bureau of Labor Statistics, U.S. Department of Labor. (2012). Social workers. *Occupational Outlook Handbook, 2012–13 Ed.* Retrieved from http://www.bls.gov/ooh/community-and-social-service/social-workers.htm

Butler, A., Ford, D., & Tregaskis, C. (2007). Who do we think we are? Self and reflexivity in social work practice. *Qualitative Social Work, 6,* 281–299.

Carey, M., & Foster, V. (2011). Social work, ideology and the limits of post-hegemony. *Journal of Social Work.* Advance online publication. doi:10.1177/1468017311412032

Cheetham, G., & Chivers, G. (2001). How professionals learn in practice: An investigation of informal learning amongst people working in professions. *Journal of European Industrial Training, 25,* 248–292.

Coffield, F. (1999). Breaking the consensus: Lifelong learning as social control. *British Educational Research Journal, 25,* 479–499.

Congress, E. P. (2012). Continuing education: Lifelong learning for social work practitioners and educators. *Journal of Social Work Education, 48,* 397–401.

Council on Social Work Education. (2008). *Educational policy and accreditation standards.* Alexandria, VA: Author. Retrieved from http://www.cswe.org/File.aspx?id=13780

Cournoyer, B. R., & Stanley, M. J. (2002). *The social work portfolio: Planning, assessing and documenting life-long learning in a dynamic profession.* Pacific Grove, CA: Brooks/Cole.

Cross, T. L., Friesen, B. J., Jivanjee, P., Gowen, K. L., Bandurranga, A., Matthew, C., & Maher, N. (2011). Defining youth success using culturally appropriate community-based participatory research methods. *Best Practices in Mental Health, 7,* 94–114.

Daley, B. J. (2001). Learning and professional practice: A study of four professions. *Adult Education Quarterly, 52,* 39–54.

Deakin-Crick, R., & Wilson, K. (2005). Being a learner: A virtue for the 21st century. *British Journal of Educational Studies, 53,* 359–374.

Feit, M. D. (2003). Toward a definition of social work practice: Reframing the dichotomy. *Research on Social Work Practice, 13,* 357–365.

Frost, N. (2001). Professionalism, change and the politics of lifelong learning. *Studies in Continuing Education, 23,* 5–17.

Gambrill, E. (2006). *Social work practice: A critical thinker's guide.* New York, NY: Oxford University Press.

Gardiner, H. P., & Kline, T. J. B. (2007). Development of the employee lifelong learning scale. *PAACE Journal of Lifelong Learning, 16,* 63–72.

Gibbs, L., & Gambrill, E. (2002). Evidence-based practice: Counterarguments to objections. *Research on Social Work Practice, 12*, 452–476.

Goldman, E. (2009). Learning in a chaotic environment. *Journal of Workplace Learning, 21*, 555–574.

Gustavsson, B. (2002). What do we mean by lifelong learning and knowledge? *International Journal of Lifelong Education, 21*, 13–23.

Hackett, S. (2001). Educating for competency and reflective practice: Fostering a conjoint approach in education and training. *Journal of Workplace Learning, 13*, 103–112.

Hare, I. (2004). Defining social work for the 21st century: The International Federation of Social Workers' revised definition of social work. *International Social Work, 47*, 407–424.

Hawkins, L., Fook, J., & Ryan, M. (2001). Social workers' use of the language of social justice. *British Journal of Social Work, 31*, 1–13.

Holosko, M. J. (2003). The history of the working definition of practice. *Research on Social Work Practice, 13*, 271–283.

Huang, L. N., Hepburn, K. S., & Espiritu, R. C. (2003). To be or not to be . . . evidence based? *Data Matters, 6*, 1–3.

Isaacs, M. R., Huang, L. N., Hernandez, M., & Echo-Hawk, H. (2005). *The road to evidence: The intersection of evidence-based practices and cultural competence in children's mental health*. Washington, DC: National Association of Multi-Ethnic Behavioral Health Associations.

Jarvis, P. (2006). Beyond the learning society: Globalization and the moral imperative for reflective social change. *International Journal of Lifelong Education, 25*, 201–211.

Jones, L., & Moore, R. (1993). Education, competence, and the control of expertise. *British Journal of the Sociology of Education, 14*, 385–397.

Kadushin, A., & Harkness, D. (2002). *Supervision in social work* (4th ed.). New York, NY: Columbia University Press.

Kasworm, C., & Hemminsen, L. (2007). Preparing professionals for lifelong learning: Comparative examination of master's education programs. *Higher Education, 54*, 449–468.

Kirby, J. R., Knapper, C., Lamon, P. & Eganoff, W. J. (2010). Developemnt of a scale to measure lifelong learning. *International Journal of Lifelong Education, 29*, 291–302.

Knowles, M. (1990). *The adult learner: A neglected species* (4th ed.). Houston, TX: Gulf.

Lam, D. O. B., Wong, D. K. P., Hui, H. S. K., Lee, F. W. L, & Chan, E. K. L. (2006). Preparing social workers to be lifelong learners. *Journal of Teaching in Social Work, 26*, 103–119.

Leslie, D. R., & Cassano, R. (2003). The working definition of social work practice: Does it work? *Research on Social Work Practice, 13*, 366–375.

Lester, S. (1995). Beyond knowledge and competence: Towards a framework for professional education. *Capability, 1*, 1–12.

Lewis, M. (1998). Lifelong learning: Why professionals must have the desire for and the capacity to continue learning throughout life. *Health Information Management, 28*, 62–66.

Lowery, C. T. (1998). American Indian perspectives on addiction and recovery. *Health and Social Work, 23*, 127–135.

McBeath, B., Briggs, H., & Aisenberg, E. (2010). Examining the premises supporting the empirically supported intervention approach to social work practice. *Social Work, 55*, 347–357.

Morgan-Klein, B., & Osborne, M. (2007). *The concepts and practices of lifelong learning*. London, UK: Routledge.

National Association of Social Workers. (2012). *Social work profession*. Retrieved from http://www.naswdc.org/pressroom/features/general/profession.asp

Olssen, M. (2006). Understanding the mechanisms of neoliberal control: Lifelong learning, flexibility and knowledge capitalism. *International Journal of Lifelong Education, 25*, 213–230.

Panda, M., & Desbiens, N. (2010). An "education for life" requirement to promote lifelong learning in an internal residency program. *Journal for Graduate Medical Education, 12*, 562–565.

Parrish, D. E., & Rubin, A. (2011). An effective model for continuing education training in evidence-based practice. *Research on Social Work Practice, 21*, 77–87.

Parton, N. (2008). Changes in the form of knowledge in social work: From the 'social' to the 'informational?' *British Journal of Social Work, 38*, 253–269.

Peet, M., Lonn, S., Gurin, P., Boyer, P., Matney, M., Marra, T., . . . Daley, A. (2011). Fostering integrative knowledge through eportfolios. *International Journal of ePortfolio, 1*, 11–31.

Petracchi, H., & Zastrow, C. (2010a). Suggestions for utilizing the 2008 EPAS in CSWE-accredited Baccalaureate and Masters curriculums—Reflections from the field, Part 1: The explicit curriculum. *Journal of Teaching in Social Work, 30*, 125–146.

Petracchi, H. E., & Zastrow, C. (2010b). Suggestions for utilizing the 2008 EPAS in CSWE-accredited Baccalaureate and Masters curriculums—Reflections from the field, Part 2: The implicit curriculum. *Journal of Teaching in Social Work, 30*, 357–366.

Powell, W. W., & Snellman, K. (2004). The knowledge economy. *Annual Review of Sociology, 30*, 199–220.

Proctor, E. K. (2007). Implementing evidence-based practice in social work education: Principles, strategies, and partnerships. *Research on Social Work Practice, 17*, 583–591.

Randall, G. E., & Kindiak, D. H. (2008). Deprofessionalization or postprofessionalization? Reflections on the state of social work as a profession. *Social Work in Health Care, 47*, 341–354.

Reisch, M. (2011). *Being a radical social worker in reactionary times*. Keynote Address to the 25th Anniversary Conference of the Social Welfare Alliance, Washington, DC.

Risler, E., Lowe, L. A., & Nackerud, L. (2003). Defining social work: Does the working definition work today? *Research on Social Work Practice, 13*, 299–309.

Schoen, D. A. (1982). *The reflective practitioner: How professionals think in action*. New York, NY: HarperCollins.

Schoen, D. A. (1987). *Educating the reflective practitioner: Toward a new design for teaching and learning in the professions*. San Francisco, CA: Jossey-Bass.

Schram, S. F., & Silverman, B. (2011). *The end of social work: The neoliberalization of doing good*. Paper presented at the annual meeting of the American Political Science Association. Retrieved from http://ssrn.com/abstract=1901020

Senge, P. (1990). *The fifth discipline*. New York, NY: Currency Doubleday.

Slaton, A. E. (2003). A family perspective on evidence-based practices. *Data Matters, 6*, 17–23.

Smith, C. A., Cahoen-Callow, A., Dia, D. A., Bliss, D. L., Gantt, A., Cornelius, L. J., & Harrington, D. (2006). Staying current in a changing profession: Evaluating perceived change resulting from continuing professional education. *Journal of Social Work Education, 42*, 465–482.

Staniforth, B., Fouché, C., & O'Brien, M. (2011). Still doing what we do: Defining social work in the 21st century. *Journal of Social Work, 11*, 191–208.

Taylor, I. (1997). *Developing learning in professional education: Partnerships for practice*. London, UK: The Society for Research into Higher Education and Open University Press.

Wain, K. (2000). The learning society: Postmodern politics. *International Journal of Lifelong Learning, 28*, 62–66.

Walker, J. S., Briggs, H. E., Koroloff, N., & Friesen, B. J. (2007). Implementing and sustaining evidence-based practice in social work. *Journal of Social Work Education, 43*, 361–375.

Walters, S. (2010). 'The planet will not survive if it's not a learning planet': Sustainable development within learning through life. *International Journal of Lifelong Education, 29*, 427–436.

Walters, S. (2012). Focusing on the heart. Lifelong, life-wide, and life-deep learning in the time of HIV/AIDS. In D. N. Aspin, J. Chapman, K. Evans, & R. Bagnall (Eds.), *Second international handbook of lifelong learning, Vol. 26* (pp. 195–208). Dordrecht, The Netherlands: Springer.

Yang, B., Watkins, K. E., & Marsick, V. J. (2004). The construction of the learning organization: Dimensions, measurement and validation. *Human Resource Development Quarterly, 15*, 31–55.

Yeo, R. K. (2005). Revisiting the roots of the learning organization: A synthesis of the learning organization literature. *The Learning Organization, 12*, 368–382.

Zeira, A., & Rosen, A. (2000). Unraveling "tacit knowledge": What social workers do and why they do it. *Social Service Review, 74*, 103–122.

Social Work Continuing Education: A Statewide Case Study

Mark Gianino, Betty J. Ruth, and Scott Miyake Geron

ABSTRACT

This article presents findings from a 2013 qualitative study of social work continuing education (CE) in Massachusetts. Eleven focus groups were conducted with 75 participants from key stakeholder groups: practitioners, educators, licensing board members, and agency administrators. Although positive perspectives surfaced—such as diversity of CE options—thematic analysis nonetheless reflected considerable frustration with the current system. CE concerns included lack of access, cost, missing CE content areas, quality control issues, and lack of employer support. Participants also noted the need for enhanced transfer of CE-derived knowledge and skills in the workplace. Greater attention to this crucial aspect of professional development is therefore needed.

Introduction

Social work continuing education (CE) is a multidimensional professional issue of significant concern to a wide variety of stakeholders within and beyond the social work profession. Common to most established professions, CE serves many important functions. It is considered essential for promoting professional competence, career development, regulatory compliance, and a profession's overall well-being. Through CE, practitioners enhance professional identification, gain skills and knowledge, connect with other professionals, and fulfill licensing-related CE requirements (Strom-Gottfried, 2008). More broadly, CE facilitates knowledge translation and dissemination of best practices, with the larger goal of improving social work outcomes (McWilliam, 2007; Smith et al., 2006). This, in turn, strengthens the public perception of the profession's effectiveness and enhances its status (Dia, Smith, Cohen-Callow, & Bliss, 2005). CE is an essential component of professional lifelong learning, and support for CE is integrated into the National Association of Social Workers (NASW) Code of Ethics (NASW, 2009a; Nissen, Pendell, Jivanjee, & Goodluck, 2014), which also has established continuing education standards to guide its members. Meanwhile, CE programming and authorization are an important source of income for NASW and for many other organizations (Congress, 2012; NASW, 2009b).

Formal social work CE developed in the mid-20th century, fueled by the professionalization of social work, with initial support from schools of social work and from federal funding for social work education. As regulation of social work progressed, CE requirements eventually were linked to licensure, and individual practitioners were mandated to accrue approved CE units (CEU) for relicensure (Strom-Gottfried, 2008). Today, all jurisdictions require social work licensure or registration, and most mandate CE—usually in the form of CEU "contact hours"—to maintain licensure (Congress, 2012; Tian, Atkinson, Portnoy, & Gold, 2007).

Social work CE may include a wide array of formal educational activities including workshops, conferences, in-service trainings, webinars, certificate programs, journal or other professional reading groups, and consultative activities (Smith et al., 2006; Strom-Gottfried, 2008). Nationally, numerous entities have a stake in social work CE. Practitioners, educators, regulators, employers, and CE providers all interface with the complex world of CE, yet many of these stakeholders are unfamiliar with the complexity and depth of the issue.

Literature Review and Current Context

Although research on social work CE is limited, there are three discernible areas of inquiry. First, there are growing efforts to evaluate individual CE programs. For example, recent peer-reviewed articles focus on CE programming in areas such as military social work, supervision, evidence-based practice, and ethics in health settings (McCormick et al., 2014; Parrish & Rubin, 2011; Smith & Cheung, 2015; Smith-Osborne, 2015). These efforts reflect the growing acceptance of CE as a research topic and provide some indication of current practice areas that appear to require targeted CE. Second, since 2009, teams associated with *Professional Development: The International Journal of Continuing Social Work Education* have conducted regular surveys of social work CE, providing a useful baseline of information on the state of university-sponsored social work CE programs (Cochran & Landuyt, 2010; Landuyt & Morgan, 2014). Finally, a few scholars have attempted the difficult task of studying aspects of CE effectiveness. Studies have focused on the development of a CE evaluation instrument (Coyle & Carter, 2011), the examination of perceived motivation for CE participation (Dia et al., 2005), assessment of how CE affects professional identity (Valutis, Rubin, & Bell, 2012), and evaluation of perceived changes in knowledge and skill as a result of participation in CE (Smith et al., 2006). Although the emerging research base is useful, there are significant gaps. These include the absence of a national perspective on stakeholders' experiences with CE, lack of research on the effectiveness of different modes of CE, little understanding of how CE impacts social work outcomes over time, and uncertainty whether participation in CE actually achieves its goal of enhancing practice competence (Daley, 2001; Gianino, Geron, Sheehan, & Ruth, 2014; Strom-Gottfried, 2008).

A review of the multifaceted issues that surrounds CE provides additional context for appreciating the growing concerns.

Growth

The profession is growing; with more than 600,000 professional social workers, it clearly is now the dominant mental health profession in the country (NASW, 2015). The U.S. Bureau of Labor Statistics predicts the demand for social workers will increase 19% from 2012–2022 (Bureau of Labor Statistics, 2014). Accompanying this growth are increasing pressures to demonstrate the profession's competence in mastering emerging knowledge and skills, particularly the use of empirically supported interventions and outcomes (Davenport & Wodarski, 1989; Kirk & Reid, 2002; Parrish & Rubin, 2011).

The Changing Workforce

Social workers, like all workers, are living longer, changing jobs more frequently, and routinely encountering the need for new expertise in rapidly changing work environments (Ruth & Geron, 2009). Moreover, the agency context also is changing: Community-based care is replacing institutional care, evidence-based interventions are supplanting tradition-bound ones, and high tech is replacing low tech in all elements of the workplace. To meet these unprecedented demographic, service delivery and technological changes, a greater emphasis on workforce development and effective and accessible social work CE are needed (Geron, Andrews, & Kuhn, 2005; Whitaker & Arrington, 2008).

CE and Social Work Higher Education

The relationship of social work CE to social work higher education is varied and ambivalent, and it is difficult to discern whether schools of social work view CE as relevant to their mission (Ruth & Geron, 2009). In their biennial study of school of social work–based CE programs, Landuyt and Morgan (2014) noted that there is little coordination among CE programs nationally; it appears that some schools of social work simply do not offer CE and that many programs limp along with few staff and little funding from their host institutions. This finding may be due to general changes in social work education. As has been widely observed, social work faculty—particularly at top-tier schools—are increasingly focused on research, not practice; furthermore, many new faculty members have had fewer than 2 years of post-MSW practice experience prior to embarking on careers as social work educators (Johnson & Munch, 2010). A significant number of faculty members are unlicensed and therefore may be disconnected from experiences of regulation and CE; still others may view licensure as controversial or irrelevant to them (Marson, 2006; Thyer, 2007).

Yet several signs point to a renewed academy interest in CE. The Council on Social Work Education (CSWE), the accrediting body for BSW and MSW programs, now includes language in its Educational Policy and Accreditation Standards promoting professional development and lifelong learning (CSWE, 2015). The evidence-based practice movement may be another important driver, even though a growing body of research suggests that practicing social workers rarely read research, evaluate their own practice, or utilize empirically supported interventions (Parrish & Rubin, 2011). Nevertheless, CE is emerging as an important tool in decreasing the research/practice gap, and as such is garnering increased attention from the academy (Rubin & Parrish, 2007).

Regulation as a Driver of CE Concern

CE participation is required for license renewal in almost all jurisdictions, and regulators therefore have an important stake in knowing if, how, and under what circumstances CE is effective in enhancing practice competence and protecting the public interest (Bibus & Boutte-Queen, 2011). From a regulatory point of view, the burden for obtaining CE lies squarely with the practitioner; still, the Association of Social Work Boards (ASWB) recognizes the centrality of quality control and attempts to educate practitioners on how to evaluate program quality. To that end, it has promulgated standards for quality CE and created an authorizing entity that approves high-quality CE (ASWB, 2011). Nevertheless, it is generally acknowledged that quality control across the field is uneven, standards for the evaluation of CE are lacking, and CE requirements vary significantly by state (Mansouri & Lockyer, 2007). Moreover, there is some evidence that the types of CE routinely approved by licensing boards, such as conferences and workshops, do not reflect the needs of adult learners and may not result in practice behavior changes or improved work performance (Howard, McMillan, & Pollio, 2003). Although the current model of "contact hours" or "continuing education units" is standard in the field, this model's effectiveness remains unknown (Daley, 2001). A vast, profitable, and largely unregulated network of competing organizations offering myriad forms of CE—from the popular celebrity speaker to the "CEU mill"—has emerged in recent years. Practitioners are left to their own devices to sort through the quality of the offerings (Ruth & Geron, 2009).

Social work CE is clearly a dense and complicated arena. A more systematic inquiry into CE is needed to determine if it is meeting its threefold goal of enhanced competence, improved practice outcomes, and public protection. Without such effort, the paucity of high-quality CE may become an issue in an otherwise successful effort to capitalize on the numerical dominance of the profession during a time of significant change and opportunity.

The Missing Link Project

In 2011, the ASWB's Foundation for Research and Consumer Education in Social Work Regulation funded a team of researchers at Boston University School of Social Work (BUSSW) to undertake a study of social work CE in North America. The Missing Link Project's (MLP's) purpose was to develop a clearer understanding of the intersecting issues related to quality and effectiveness of the current CE system and to make recommendations for improvement. MLP identified CE stakeholder groups—practitioners, educators, providers, and regulators—and sought to broadly assess each of their views, utilizing a mixed methods approach. The MLP study included two components: a structured national survey of states and Canadian provinces and an in-depth qualitative study of a single state (the Massachusetts Case Study). Findings from this state study are reported here.

Participants and Procedures

The Massachusetts Case Study employed a qualitative design to obtain a deeper, more grounded understanding of the views of stakeholders through the use of focus groups. Stakeholders were defined as all Massachusetts social work practitioners, including licensed, unlicensed, and macro practitioners; social work educators; licensing board administrators; professional organization administrators; social work students; and other key informants such as researchers, CE providers, and leaders in the Massachusetts social work community. A team of four researchers conducted a series of 11 focus groups with stakeholders across the state, beginning in January 2012 and ending in June 2013. Because of the diversity of the stakeholder groups, the methods for recruitment differed; the following discussion includes the groups conducted, their geographic location, and the sampling method used for each.

(1) Practitioner Groups: Three practitioner groups, consisting of mixed macro and micro (clinical) social workers, were recruited from across Massachusetts using the BUSSW Professional Education Program listserv, which included e-mail addresses of more than 5,000 Massachusetts social workers. Twenty-eight practitioners participated.

(2) State Board Administrators Group: Three state licensing board administrators, all social workers, participated. Unfortunately, due to legal constraints, actual board members were unable to participate.

(3) Faculty Groups: Three faculty focus groups were held across the state. The sample was collected by compiling a database of all social work faculty members from Massachusetts MSW/BSW program websites. Faculty was invited to participate in any of the three groups, and 17 participated.

(4) Macro-Group: Because macro social workers often are unlicensed in Massachusetts, it is unclear whether they participate in traditional CE. To increase the voice of this underrepresented group, we reached out to Massachusetts macro/community social workers to participate in their own homogenous group. Macro faculty, the BUSSW Associate Dean of Alumni Affairs and External Relations, and the Macro Field Director identified macro practitioners and provided e-mail addresses. We recruited from this list, and six participated.

(5) Key Informant Group: Key informants were identified as having special insight, knowledge, or experience in the profession, including having served in varied leadership roles in the state. The MLP team members, together with the BUSSW Associate Deans, helped to identify these key informants and provided e-mail addresses for them. A total of nine participated.

(6) Student Group: A cohort of 2nd-year BUSSW students participated in a student-facilitated focus group. These students were recruited via the school's student listserv, and eight participated.

(7) Massachusetts NASW: The state chapter of NASW (MA-NASW) professional social work staff members participated in a group. All staff members were invited by e-mail and by personal contact, and the group consisted of four participants.

The research team developed a common set of focus group questions regarding CE, and then additional questions were added based on the particular characteristics of the stakeholders. Examples of sample questions included the following: What are your best/worst experiences with CE? From which types of CE do you learn best? What are the strengths of the current CE system? What challenges/obstacles/problems do you have regarding CE? How can CE be improved?

The MLP research study was reviewed and approved by the Boston University Institutional Review Board.

Analysis

Groups met for approximately 90 minutes and were facilitated by two team members experienced in qualitative research. Audiotapes of the sessions were professionally transcribed and thematically analyzed, using Atlas.ti.6.2 (2011), by a team of one researcher and two graduate social work students. The data analysis was informed by grounded theory in order to gain in-depth understanding of varied stakeholder experiences and views of CE. The analysis began with a read-through of each transcript, multiple times, followed by an inductive stage of open coding (Charmaz, 2006; Glaser & Strauss, 1967) in which team members worked independently on the same transcribed focus group interview responses to create initial codes. Memo writing was employed throughout the analytic process to document coding decisions (Charmaz, 2006). Team members met to compare and contrast initial codes, then group similar codes under more general categories, and finally label initial common themes. Negative case analytic methods (Padgett, 1998) were deployed to "bookmark" discrepant cases, which were noted during the analysis. These procedures were repeated with each transcription, and the team returned to previous data to refine the coding scheme. Transcripts were reviewed using axial coding (Charmaz, 2006; LaRossa, 2005; Miles & Huberman, 1994), which was additionally refined, with relevant quotes extracted. In the final stage of analysis, senior members of the MLP team reread the transcripts and evaluated the coding scheme against the data.

Results

Eight significant themes emerged from the analysis: (a) diverse motivations for CE engagement; (b) consumer experiences in the search for CE opportunities; (c) facilitators and barriers in accessing CE; (d) participant assessment of CE quality; (e) participant perception of CE effectiveness, as defined by translation of knowledge and skills into practice; (f) participant assessment of CE system strengths; (g) participant views on the weaknesses of CE; and (h) participant suggestions for improving CE.

Theme 1: Participant Motivations for CE Engagement

Across groups, there was general agreement that social workers primarily were motivated to participate in CE to fulfill the licensure maintenance mandate. Second, participants from practitioner groups spoke of their commitment to improving practice knowledge and skills; for many participants, CE, in fact, was a job requirement. Finally, a number of practitioners indicated that they were motivated by a search for personal or professional enrichment, often seeking new knowledge outside their current role or area of focus.

Theme 2: Consumer Search for CE Opportunities

A number of striking observations were made by participants regarding the search for CE. In general, informants described a highly individualistic process that greatly depended on the motivation of the individual practitioner. There was no reliable way to access information on CE, and participants frequently spoke of being bombarded by marketing flyers and online invitations to CE, few of which they could assess for quality. According to one informant: "You get all these flyers, now it's two for one, or buy two, get one free, or whatever, and I'm like what does that even mean? What's the quality here?" Some informants observed that agencies generally did not assist practitioners in locating quality, affordable CE opportunities. Several commented on the need for an online review site (like Yelp) that would offer consumer assessments of CE presenters and programs. One practitioner observed simply, "A presenter rating system would be helpful. Like, I can go online before I buy a car, I can do a comparison shop."

Many participants spoke of tending to go with a "known brand," or making assumptions about quality based on the name recognition of the presenter, or the credibility of the sponsoring institution. Some observed that CE consumers seem to seek out "hot topics" and popular, but not necessarily effective, methods. According to one faculty participant,

> I've been told when I've wanted to give presentations that people are (only) really interested in cognitive behavioral therapy … they're not going to come to something if it's about the intersection of gender and race, or sexual orientation and race, and that strikes me as interesting given our profession and given what we say we do. (SW Faculty)

Theme 3: Facilitators and Barriers in Accessing CE

Even after identifying appropriate CE, practitioners spoke about significant barriers to participation. The most commonly noted one was cost: Numerous informants indicated that, as agencies reduce funding for continuing education, social workers are required to pay more out of pocket. Speaking to this frustration, one noted:

> In my organization they have (so few) professional development funds that you have to put in this lengthy application about why you want to go, how it's going to connect to your job, and make you better at your job. And I don't want to write an essay about this just to get $100 because I'm already busy enough. So sometimes those things fall off the plate because I would have to put in extra work to make it happen, or pay for it myself out of my own pocket. (Practitioner)

Practitioners engaged in private clinical practice were especially vocal. "When you're self-employed in private practice, you have to pay for everything yourself. Not easy." Many participants described making tradeoffs between quality and cost—usually selecting the cheapest CEs, even though they generally were perceived as being of the lowest quality. Other barriers related to the required, but often uncompensated, time off from work associated with CE. Numerous stakeholders observed that agencies' commitments here had diminished, as reflected in the lack of funding for CE. A cogent expression of this theme was offered by one board regulator:

> I think the days of agencies paying for their employees to take CE and providing CE for their employees are pretty few and far between. Licensees are seeing that the agencies are feeling this push for productivity, and to make money, and that agencies have kind of lost the value of continuing education. … It's always been so interesting to me that here are these agencies that are employing these licensees

and requiring that these people have a license to work at their agency because you're going to get more money when they get reimbursed if this person is licensed, yet they're not willing to provide them with what they need to maintain that license, be it supervision or CE. It has really always been very annoying and sad to me that this is the state of things in most settings where our licensees are employed. (Board Regulator)

Finally, other barriers include lack of accessibility of various CE locations, including adequate parking, public transportation, and settings inaccessible for people with disabilities.

Theme 4: Participant Assessment of CE Quality

Broad concern was expressed about CE quality across all participant groups. Informants from all our constituency groups offered rich, in-depth perspectives on this issue from their varied vantage points as board regulators, providers of CE, students, faculty, and consumers. One senior professor stated, "I've been worried over many years about the state of continuing education because it just seems so variable, and I puzzle about it as a provider and also as a recipient." CEU booklets containing printed lectures were widely criticized, with one key informant observing, "… using those blue books. They have to go because that's not doing anything to benefit us as a profession. If that's how you're getting your CEs, then quite honestly I'm not going to go to you for therapy."

Licensing board participants articulated conundrums faced in their disciplinary roles, such as when complaints are lodged—and substantiated—against social workers. Disciplinary actions, for instance, sometimes include mandated CE on topics such as ethics. Board participants noted that unfortunately, such courses often are not offered. Another area of board participant frustration was a lack of CE on record keeping—another commonly mandated area specified for remediation. Finally, board informants lamented the paucity of quality, evidence-based practice CE and were skeptical regarding most CE providers' focus instead on

> the "sexier" programs that are going to attract more licensees which may not be evidence-based practice models. They may be just the equivalent of "Basket Weaving 101," but the sponsoring entities are going to find a way to get them approved because they know that those are going to be the ones that get licensees in, and they're going to make money off of them.

Participants from NASW, a major CE provider and authorizing entity in Massachusetts, articulated similar concerns regarding highly variable CE quality. According to one NASW staff member, quality is in decline due to "more and more cheap, easy CEs, and less oversight of quality … less oversight of the presenters." The informant further observed that this reality has resulted in a proliferation of unqualified presenters and programs. NASW informants admitted that, as a nonprofit, they faced challenges on the "business side," such as the inability to pay high-quality presenters enough, acknowledging that paying more would mean that NASW "would be priced out of the market."

As consumers of CE, practitioner informants offered passionate views on the factors that contributed to, or inhibited, CE quality. There was broad agreement about (a) the importance of dynamic, interactive, and engaging presenters; (b) the role of technology in aiding or inhibiting learning, and (c) the fact that a "famous" name does not necessarily correlate with a quality learning experience. There was nearly unanimous agreement among practitioners and students that the quality of CE correlated positively with hands- on, interactive, and dynamic content delivery. One practitioner described quality as follows: "Did I feel like the presenter connected with me and the audience in some way? Were there different kinds of styles, not just lecture method, but also mixing it up a little bit. For me as a learner...that is really important."

Some student focus group members had been exposed to CE through agency trainings or agency-sponsored regional conferences. Student participants articulated the importance of their social work education in socializing them to lifelong learning. They echoed their colleagues' views that the essence of a quality program included good audience engagement and an emphasis on takeaway skills. One student participant compared the experience of a quality training to that of a good class:

> Interacting with the audience, using a visual presentation, and having handouts is important, but getting the audience really integrated in the work, asking questions perhaps, using some examples. It's kind of like when you go to class and you know which good teachers are worth it, and so it's the same with a [CE] presentation.

Several practitioner participants noted that learning is enhanced when presenters were willing to discuss cases that did not go well, illustrating lessons learned from their mistakes. According to one informant, "Their presentation was quite brave; they took apart all the mistakes that they made in their work and the way they presented it ... was really refreshing. ... I think there were 30 people in the room, and probably 28 of them were really engaged." One NASW staff participant defined quality as obtaining at least one thing that can be taken away and applied: "As a consumer, what I look for when I go to a CE program is a kernel. I want to go away with at least one new thing that I can practice, that I can think about."

As CE consumers, practitioner informants had a great deal to say about the lack of quality among some CE offerings. The greatest criticism was aimed at presenters who seemed disengaged from the audience or who merely read off slides. Informants across groups both praised and lamented the role of technology in CE. Some described frustration in attending presentations where quality was much diminished by poor technology or equipment breakdown.

Informants shared their ambivalence about online learning—both appreciating the convenience of varied formats, such as webinars and podcasts, and missing the interactive component that accompanies in-person CE. As noted, many informants told us that they selected CE on the basis of name recognition. However, they acknowledged that at times the programs did not live up to the presenters' reputations. One practitioner informant put it this way:

> You know sometimes it doesn't mean that somebody who's famous is going to be a good teacher. You sit for 8 hours and wonder what did he just say for 8 hours? This very famous big shot in the field comes (and you pay a whole lot of money) but he is not necessarily a good teacher.

Finally, many informants related that the experience of quality CE programming was linked to accuracy in advertising; participants were especially disappointed when advanced content was promised in the promotional literature, but presentations were at the beginner level.

Theme 5: Participant Perception of CE Effectiveness, as Defined by Translation of Knowledge and Skills Into Practice

Informants across all participant groups spoke about CE effectiveness. If participants conceptualized quality as the *experience* of a CE program—good presentation, accurate information, taught in a thoughtful, engaging way—then effectiveness was about what they took away that could be *applied* to practice. This perspective was succinctly summarized by one practitioner: "I like the skill-based training. I think that's important. I find that people really like to come and get something concrete that they can apply directly to their practice."

According to our informants, CE effectiveness involved an assessment that they learned content well enough to translate it into practice. Here, workplace factors proved to be of considerable importance. Predictably, participants endorsed the perspective that effectiveness was enhanced when employers supported the integration of new skills and knowledge. This conviction would be demonstrated, according to participants, when agencies provided sufficient time and support to implement their new learning into the practice setting. Respondents reported considerable variability in the commitment of employers to the integration and transfer of CE to practice. Across most groups, they also noted that effectiveness had to be linked to outcome measurement over time as they attempted to apply new skills on the job, not just simple evaluation at the end of the training. This factor was echoed by numerous practitioners: "Talk … about how you're going to integrate it, to me that's really the whole point of continuing education—learning content and then figuring out how to actually use it when you're sitting with a real live human being who is suffering. To me, that's the only point in doing it."

Several informants reported frustration when training experiences offered little to enhance their practice. This feeling of disappointment was especially true for respondents who were compelled to attend CE but found little to take back to their setting. According to one key informant,

> I did a two-day trauma training. I think trauma work is so complicated, and if you don't do it right, it is problematic, but I feel like it's a great training. I learned some valuable things. But I don't know how to implement it where I work. … If you're bringing something in that's really a specialized treatment, and your agency doesn't incorporate that type of work, I think it's really a challenge to find a way to apply it.

Several participants observed that, although new learning may not be immediately transferable, agencies can play a critical role in assisting practitioners in adapting new skills to practice. Unfortunately, most participants expressed the view that agency support frequently was lacking, and the transfer of newly learned skills was entirely left up to the individual. In the fast-paced, complex, and crisis-driven environments in which many participants were employed, there was little time for reflection and integration. Faculty informants particularly lamented the loss of attention on agency-based training, due to productivity pressures. Although the promotion of a robust learning environment at work and a commitment to productivity do not have to be antithetical, such was the experience articulated by many participants. Board respondents, in particular, expressed alarm regarding the diminishing utilization of program evaluation tools in both live programming and online CE. According to board informants, CE consumers, who may only be minimally engaged in a face-to-face training, are at least required to complete an evaluation of the program; in other formats, it is easier to check out altogether. Finally, several participants suggested that the current CE model "simply does not work" because knowledge and skills accrue over time, when there are opportunities for practice and reinforcement, and CE generally is not set up this way. According to one faculty informant,

> We know from adult education that it's the follow up that works over time, yet most continuing education isn't set up that way at all, so we already know it's not going to necessarily lead to [the mastery of new] knowledge or even to enhanced practice skills.

Although there was broad agreement that program evaluation is essential to measuring CE effectiveness, many agreed that the current system of a "one shot" end-of workshop evaluation provides scant information on quality or effectiveness. Several suggested that participants should receive CE certificates only after they provide detailed and specific feedback on their learning. According to one practitioner,

> I've gotten so many evaluations that are just like—do you feel like your knowledge was improved; like 1 through 4, what was your knowledge before this? And I'll check

that off, but that does not tell anything about what I've actually learned. I know it's a pain to write it down, but ask me to write something about what I've learned … because the 1 through 4 [Likert assessment] doesn't mean a thing.

Theme 6: Participant Assessment of CE System Strengths

Across all focus groups, participants spoke of the strengths of CE, making important observations about what was "working." These included (a) the diversity of CE, offered at a wide variety of cost, topics, and delivery models; (b) the acknowledgment that requiring CE serves as a built-in mechanism for increasing practitioner knowledge and skills; (c) the recognition that CE functions as a means of burnout prevention; and (d) the sense that CE may reduce feelings of isolation, promote connection, and create opportunities for networking. According to one macro informant, although macro CE generally represents only a small minority portion of CE offerings, its emergence is viewed as a positive factor:

> What I do think is working well is that the topic areas are so varied. I'm a macro social worker, and I think it's important to have CE programs that take that into account that macro social workers need CEs too, and we're not a specialty area. I can go to a school's social work conference but I'm going to get CE for a specialty area that's not really mine. So I think it's encouraging to see that there are more macro-focused CE programs. (Macro Practitioner)

There was nearly unanimous agreement among participants that the many formats and types of CE are a sign of strength, a view represented by this practitioner comment:

> One of the strengths of the way that CE is offered is that there are a lot of different ways you can get it. You can attend an in-person class, you can do a webinar, you can read the NASW 'Focus' and send in the thing and get one or one and a half CEs, lots of different modalities.

Informants also flagged the opportunity that CE provides to connect with others as an additional strength. From the perspective of a faculty participant, CE socializes students and new graduates to the profession and connects them to a lifelong learning community of colleagues. One faculty member noted that there was untapped potential in using CE as a translational process:

> As a researcher, I know that there are new ideas out there all the time. And even in the medical world, it takes approximately 15–17 years to get that out in the community, and that's not acceptable. So I think that another thing that continuing education can do is help us to become more effective in whatever it is that we're doing and I don't think that social workers necessarily have all the resources they need in order to facilitate that. (Faculty)

As discussed, practitioners are motivated to participate in CE for many reasons. The goal of practitioner rejuvenation and burnout prevention is a significant motive for some. One practitioner informant described that in one's workplace, a practitioner can start to "slack off ... may need to crank it back up. This is my professional role and I've just been sailing along smoothly. With CE, now I've got the fire lit again." Finally, a view endorsed by many practitioner participants was that CE functions as a vehicle for sustaining a social work learning community. Informants noted that this system worked best for them when they had an opportunity to connect with other social workers at trainings. This albeit latent function contributed to ambivalence about the current trend toward online learning; some participants were clear that the convenience of online learning for quick CEUs was appreciated, but many were concerned that use of this pathway could lead to greater isolation.

Theme 7: Participant Views on CE Weaknesses

There was extensive, energetic discussion among participants regarding continuing social work education's present weaknesses. One of the most frequent themes was that of content gaps. Informants spoke to the apparent lack of CE needs assessment and how that contributed to an apparent proliferation of presentations on popular topics rather than other much needed content. Among state board and NASW staff informants there was broad agreement that CE is market driven and that CE providers are dependent upon earning income by offering what is profitable and popular. Missing content areas were identified across many domains: social justice issues, social work profession-specific content, workplace safety, and macro offerings were cited most frequently. (Unlike some other states, Massachusetts does not require specific CE content.) Although many practitioners appreciated the freedom to participate in CE programs of their choice, there was virtually universal endorsement of the position that certain content, such as ethics and cultural competence, was too important *not* to mandate.

Predictably, board informants spoke most forcefully from a consumer protection orientation regarding the potentially negative impact of missing content, as well as the lack of accountability by authorizing entities that approve CE programs. These participants argued that if CE-related regulations were clearer, and based on explicit standards, it would enable boards to hold CE providers more accountable. According to one board informant, "The regulations are pretty basic and so it's not really setting the bar very high right now. I think that if we were able to beef up the regulations a bit it would enable us, with our very limited resources, to hold them more accountable." Comments from board informants suggested support for changing the culture of CE from one of compliance with requirements to one of a commitment to lifelong learning and public protection. This outcome might be achieved through greater collaboration with professional organizations and universities, which could assist with the evaluation of effectiveness, as well as the development of CE in less popular but crucial areas such as record keeping, confidentiality, consumer protection, and ethics. As noted, there was moderately strong endorsement across all groups that certain CE content should be required for licensure renewal. Most often, participants referenced ethics, but other content also was noted.

An interesting comment illustrated the practice–academy divide. A faculty member spoke to the challenges of preparing students for a constantly changing workforce, noting,

> What is expected in the job market is different than what we teach here. We are preparing people for generalist practice when they leave here. But that's not what the world is expecting from us. They're expecting highly skilled, highly trained people who have got at least one theoretical model fairly well mastered under their belt. … That's what I hear from field instructors.

Another faculty member observed, "We've really stayed in our silos, and CE is a really great example of what's reinforcing those silos. (We need to) figure out ways that CE (can be) cross disciplinary, intra disciplinary, and transdisciplinary as well".

Another theme that surfaced across practitioner groups was the value of supervision to ensure lifelong learning, hence a recommendation to change the regulations so that supervision would count as CE in Massachusetts. In a related observation, participants questioned the value of the CEU contact-hour model as a measure of learning. One practitioner participant suggested an alternative approach:

> One of the problems with the way things are set up now is that a CEU hour is a poor measure because it doesn't really get at the quality or effectiveness of the training. And if there was a way to assess quality or effectiveness, as a way to determine how many CEs you got, it would be a much easier way for you to figure out how to spend your time. So, if you go to a CEU mill to get quick & dirty CEUs, maybe you get fewer CEUs because it was a less valuable learning experience. But, if you go to a really super session that's 3 hours long, but it's an incredibly valuable learning experience, why not get 10 CEUs?

Theme 8: Participant Suggestions for Improving CE

Across all focus groups, respondents suggested a wide range of methods for improving the CE system. Given the complexity and broad scope of the observations, this final section highlights but a few of the participant recommendations.

CE Providers

The view that the development of quality standards for CE presenters in fact is necessary was strongly endorsed by all groups. There was further agreement that CE providers should create programs based on a systematic needs assessment. There also was strong validation of the need for affordable and accessible CE programs to ensure continued vitality and viability of social work CE. One practitioner participant put it this way:

> I think I would make it so that quality CE was financially affordable and accessible to everyone. I mean, for social workers who just started out and who make $28,000 a year, they're going to go and get the $3.99 CEUs. They eat Ramen Noodles, I mean, that's what's going to happen.

Board Regulators

One CE provider participant stated simply, "I would like policing and standardization from the board regarding approval of CEs, set(ting) a standard that's across the field." A strong endorsement for requiring ethics content was reflected in the following comment from a board administrator:

> I think we would all agree that a requirement of at least 3 CEUs in ethics would be huge, and would certainly be something that we would recommend that the board truly consider in any move to a regulation change.

Another board participant recommended a rotation of required topics over multiple licensing renewal cycles. Finally, a central theme that surfaced across practitioner groups was the value of supervision and mentoring for lifelong learning and hence a recommendation that CE regulations be amended so that approved supervision could count as some portion of CE.

Schools of Social Work

Faculty participants noted that there was an opportunity to claim CE as a focal area for schools of social work and endorsed the need to support CE as part of higher education's service to the profession. One faculty participant suggested that schools could facilitate conversations among diverse constituencies to drive a research-to-practice agenda that values stakeholder voices:

> What I see happening in our program is that continuing education is very faculty-driven, and it's really based on faculty perceptions about what practitioners need. I tend to be more of a bottom up kind of person myself. I would like to see us do more partnerships with agencies and communities to have all of the stakeholders' voices be heard in planning continuing education so that we're giving people what they need, and maybe some of what we think they need, but that *their* needs are driving what we're providing, rather than vice versa.

Role of Employers

In addition to supporting their employees' participation in CE, agencies were urged to consider how to help practitioners utilize what they learn. Among participants, there was strong endorsement of the idea that agencies do more to both support social workers' attendance at CE programs and to educate supervisors about how to facilitate the translation of supervisees' new learning and skills into practice:

> Translating what you hear, what you see in a conference and bringing it back to work, asking: How often did you use this skill? How effective was this skill? What did you learn from this skill? And what can you now do differently? (Practitioner)

Role of Professional Organizations

One practitioner participant suggested that NASW should take the lead in establishing a process for vetting the quality of CE across the confusing array of proliferating entities by creating a free, centralized rating system.

Discussion

The MLP's Massachusetts Case Study provides insight into stakeholder views and experiences of CE in one state. The study, which drew participants from across the Commonwealth, gives a rich description of the concerns, best practices, experiences, and obstacles experienced by stakeholders as they sought to provide, regulate, or obtain CE. The voices of practitioners, both micro and macro, are particularly illuminating and suggest deep frustration with the current system. Although strengths were noted—including breadth of offerings and diversity of topics—participants voiced many concerns, ranging from access, cost and missing content areas, quality control concerns, lack of employer support, and the need for an enhanced transfer of knowledge and skills to professional practice. The loneliness and individual burden felt by many social workers, as they sought to identify, purchase, and learn from CE, was particularly poignant, as was their disappointment when (not infrequently) expensive CE did not meet their needs. Other cohorts, such as faculty, board administrators, and professional organization staff, also expressed concerns regarding how best to support and enhance the CE experience. Certain worries were common across groups: Cost, access, quality, effectiveness, and skills transfer were universal.

Limitations

As with any study that draws from one geographical area, the views, experiences, and perspectives of the participants in the Massachusetts Case Study may not necessarily be shared by CE stakeholders in other states. Massachusetts is unique given the vast number of institutions of higher education per capita and the many CE programs available to residents. (Even within the state, which includes large cities and equally large rural areas, the findings are not generalizable.) Despite the researchers' efforts to recruit broadly, the majority of participants—with the exception of social work faculty stakeholder groups—hailed from the greater Boston area. Finally, it is possible that those who responded to an invitation to participate in a discussion about CE are different from the universe of social workers, perhaps more interested or discontented. Despite such limitations, this Massachusetts Case Study would appear to be the first of its kind to inquire into the views of diverse social work CE stakeholders. We very much hope that this study will make a modest contribution to the small, but growing, base of research on social work continuing education.

Implications

The findings from this study suggest that constituents broadly understand the importance of CE to the profession and to the public. Although findings indicated that all stakeholder groups are concerned about CE quality and effectiveness, most are not in dialogue with one another about how to address the issues and conundrums embedded in this arena. Like the story about three blind men in a room with an elephant, each of whom describes an ear, a tail, and a trunk without having a full grasp of the elephant, the respondents in our study, although informed by their own perspectives, had scant understanding of the views or mandates of the other stakeholders. Although there appears to be a degree of consensus on several issues, there was also a sense of disconnect among the stakeholders, with practitioners particularly eager for the profession "to do something" about the present state of CE as they experienced it as mandated consumers.

The current social work CE environment cannot properly be called a system. Efforts are needed to organize what is, at present, a mixed and random array of offerings of varying quality and unknown effectiveness. Each stakeholder group has a vested interest and hence a role to play in CE improvement. Clearly, profession-wide leadership is needed to ignite a broad conversation about the importance of CE and to form an action plan for large-scale improvements. As a first step, the profession can make CE a more visible issue. Leadership is needed from CSWE, NASW, and the National Association of Social Work Deans and Directors. These major organizations, for example, can create special initiatives to investigate and promote linkage of the academy to CE research. National conferences can feature additional sessions on this subject, and the National Association of Social Work Deans and Directors, CSWE, and the Society for Social Work Research could generate research interest by promoting CE dissertation research and investigation. Principal investigators can be encouraged to "write CE into" major grants so that CE becomes linked to best practices research. Other social work journals can create special calls for CE papers, such as the call here by the *Journal of Teaching in Social Work*, featuring specific CE practice areas such as gerontology, health, or child welfare. Social work regulators, together with ASWB, can continue to further promote the positive role regulation can play in improving practitioner effectiveness and public protection. Major professional organizations, such as NASW, can collaborate with researchers and regulators to formulate a validated ranking system for CE quality and a standardized policy of authorization. Finally, practitioners themselves can be encouraged to participate in national conversations about CE and to provide systemic feedback. As is evidenced in this one-state study, many of the best suggestions for improving CE came from practitioners endeavoring to meet their professional development needs via the current system.

Continuing professional education is not merely an issue of compliance with licensure requirements, although that is an important motivation for participation. CE today fulfills numerous functions in the profession, although not as completely or as effectively as it could. Although the current CE system may be a weak or "missing link" in social work professionalism, it need not remain that way. CE can become a major conduit for connecting social work research to practice. Beyond basic knowledge and skills building, CE can promote engagement in lifelong learning, professional identity development and cohesion, and networking opportunities. These in turn will likely help with retention, burnout prevention, and workforce stabilization. CE, done well, can assist the profession in examining its effectiveness, measuring practice outcomes, and furthering the science of social work. A well-established CE system, with clear quality controls, can make professional life easier for practitioners and attract employers who will have good reason to have added confidence in the social workforce. It has been said that the "great aim" of education is not merely knowledge but action (Spencer, 1894). If social work's "great aim" is to reduce human suffering and to improve human well-being, a robust and effective system of continuing professional education is an important component of our ability to ensure that we achieve our aim as a profession.

References

Association of Social Work Boards. (2011). *Continuing education advice for social workers.* Retrieved from http://www.aswb.org/education/advice/

ATLAS/ti. Version 6.2. [Computer sofware]. (2011). Berlin, Germany: Scientific Sofware Development.

Bibus, A., & Boutte-Queen, N. (2011). *Regulating social work: A primer on licensing practice.* Chicago, IL: Lyceum.

Bureau of Labor Statistics, U.S. Department of Labor. (2014). *Occupational outlook handbook, 2014-2015.* Retrieved from http://www.bls.gov/ooh/community-and-social-service/social-workers.htm

Charmaz, K. (2006). *Constructing grounded theory: A practical guide through qualitative analysis.* London, UK: Sage.

Cochran, G., & Landuyt, N. (2010). A survey of continuing education programs conducted. Professional development. *The International Journal of Continuing Social Work Education, 13*(2), 55–72.

Congress, E. P. (2012). Continuing education: Lifelong learning for social work practitioners and educators. *Journal of Social Work Education, 48*(3), 397–401. doi:10.5175/JSWE.2012.201200085

Council on Social Work Education. (2015). *Educational Policy and Accreditation Standards.* Retrieved from http://www.cswe.org/File.aspx?id=13780

Coyle, J. P., & Carter, I. (2011). Can continuing education curricula effectively teach professionals? A case for using a curriculum assessment tool for initial and ongoing evaluation. *Professional Development: International Journal of Continuing Social Work Education, 14*(1), 19–26.

Daley, B. (2001). Learning and professional practice: A study of four professions. *Adult Education Quarterly, 52*(1), 39–54. doi:10.1177/074171360105200104

Davenport, J., & Wodarski, J. S. (1989). Social work continuing education: An historical description. *Arete, 14*(1), 32–45.

Dia, D., Smith, C. A., Cohen-Callow, A., & Bliss, D. L. (2005). The education participation scale–modified: Evaluating a measure of continuing education. *Research on Social Work Practice, 15*(3), 213–222. doi:10.1177/1049731504273543

Geron, S. M., Andrews, C., & Kuhn, K. (2005). Infusing aging skills into the social work practice community: A new look at strategies for continuing professional education. *Families in Society: The Journal of Contemporary Social Services, 86*(3), 431–440. doi:10.1606/1044-3894.3442

Gianino, M., Geron, S. M., Sheehan, D., & Ruth, B. J. (2014, October). *A crisis in social work continuing professional education? A faculty conversation.* Council on Social Work Education, Annual Program Meeting, Tampa, FL.

Glaser, B., & Strauss, A. (1967). *The discovery of grounded theory.* Chicago, IL: Aldine.

Howard, M. O., McMillan, C. J., & Pollio, D. E. (2003). Teaching evidence-based practice: Toward a new paradigm for social work education. *Research on Social Work Practice, 13*, 234–259. doi:10.1177/1049731502250404

Johnson, Y. M., & Munch, S. (2010). Faculty with practice experience: The new dinosaurs in the social work academy? *Journal of Social Work Education, 46*(1), 57–66. doi:10.5175/JSWE.2010.200800050

Kirk, S. A., & Reid, W. J. (2002). *Science and social work: A critical appraisal.* New York, NY: Columbia University Press.

Landuyt, N., & Morgan, M. (2014). A survey of continuing educations programs conducted by professional development. *The International Journal of Continuing Social Work Education, 17*(1), 46–60.

LaRossa, R. (2005). Grounded theory methods and qualitative family research. *Journal of Marriage and Family, 67*, 837–857. doi:10.1111/j.1741-3737.2005.00179.x

Mansouri, M., & Lockyer, J. (2007). A meta-analysis of continuing medical education effectiveness. *Journal of Continuing Education in the Health Professions, 27*(1), 6–15. doi:10.1002/chp.88

Marson, S. (2006). Licensing of social work faculty: An issue of ethics? *Journal of Social Work Values and Ethics, 3*, 2.

McCormick, A. J., Stowell-Weiss, P., Carson, J., Tebo, G., Hanson, I., & Quesada, B. (2014). Continuing education in ethical decision making Using case studies from medical social work. *Social Work in Health Care, 53*(4), 344–363. doi:10.1080/00981389.2014.884042

McWilliam, C. L. (2007). Continuing education at the cutting edge: Promoting transformative knowledge translation. *Journal of Continuing Education in the Health Professions, 27*(2), 72–79. doi:10.1002/chp.102

Miles, M. B., & Huberman, A. M. (1994). *Qualitative data analysis: An expanded sourcebook* (2nd ed.). Thousand Oaks, CA: Sage.

National Association of Social Workers. (2015). *Social work profession*. Retrieved from http://www.socialworkers.org/pressroom/features/general/profession.asp

National Association of Social Workers. (2009a). *Code of ethics*. Retrieved from http://www.naswdc.org/pubs/code/code.asp

National Association of Social Workers. (2009b). *Continuing education*. Retrieved from http://socialworkers.org/practice/standards/cont_professional_ed.asp

Nissen, L., Pendell, K., Jivanjee, P., & Goodluck, C. (2014). Lifelong learning in social work education: A review of the literature and implications for the future. *Journal of Teaching in Social Work, 34*, 384–400. doi:10.1080/08841233.2014.936577

Padgett, D. K. (1998). Does the glove really fit? Qualitative research and clinical social work practice. *Social Work, 43*(4), 373–381. doi:10.1093/sw/43.4.373

Parrish, D. E., & Rubin, A. (2011). An effective model for continuing education training in evidence-based practice. *Research on Social Work Practice, 21*(1), 77–87. doi:10.1177/1049731509359187

Rubin, A., & Parrish, D. (2007). Challenges to the future of evidence-based practice in social work education. *Journal of Social Work Education, 43*, 405–428. doi:10.5175/JSWE.2007.200600612

Ruth, B. J., & Geron, S. M. (2009, October). *The missing link: Social work's need to strengthen continuing professional education*. Council on Social Work Education, Annual Program Meeting, San Antonio, TX.

Smith, C. A., Cohen-Callow, A., Dia, D. A., Bliss, D. L., Gantt, A., Cornelius, L. J., & Harrington, D. (2006). Staying current in a changing profession: Evaluating perceived change resulting from continued professional education. *Journal of Social Work Education, 42*(3), 465–482. doi:10.5175/JSWE.2006.042310002

Smith, D. S., & Cheung, M. (2015). Research note—Globalization and social work: Influencing practice through continuing education. *Journal of Social Work Education, 51*(3), 583–594.

Smith-Osborne, A. (2015). An intensive continuing education initiative to train social workers for military social work practice. *Journal of Social Work Education, 51*(Suppl. 1), S89–S101.

Spencer, H. (1894). *Education: Intellectual, moral, and physical*.

Strom-Gottfried, K.J. (2008). Continuing education. In T. Mizrahi and L. Davis, (eds.), *Encyclopedia of Social Work (20th ed)*. Vol. 1. New York: National Association of Social Workers, Oxford University Press.

Thyer, B. A. (2007). Social work education and clinical learning: Towards evidence-based practice? *Clinical Social Work Journal, 35*(1), 25–32. doi:10.1007/s10615-006-0064-2

Tian, J., Atkinson, N., Portnoy, B., & Gold, R. S. (2007). A systematic review of evaluation in formal continuing medical education. *Journal of Continuing Education in the Health Professions, 27*(1), 16–27. doi:10.1002/chp.89

Valutis, S., Rubin, D., & Bell, M. (2012). Professional socialization and social work values: Who are we teaching? *Social Work Education: The International Journal, 31*(8), 1046–1057. doi:10.1080/02615479.2011.610785

Whitaker, T., & Arrington, P. (2008). *Professional development. NASW membership workforce study*. Washington, DC: National Association of Social Workers.

Lessons From a New Continuing Education Mandate: The Experience of NASW-NYC

Robert Schachter

ABSTRACT

The New York City Chapter of the National Association of Social Workers (NASW-NYC), one of the largest in the country, launched a continuing education initiative in 2015 in response to passage of a new statute mandating that all MSW-level state licensed social workers begin accumulating approved hours of continuing education as a requirement for triennial licensure renewal. This article presents the NASW-NYC Chapter's response, along with the results of a participant evaluation of the conference launched by NASW-NYC to meet this new professional need.

Introduction

On January 1, 2015, a New York State statutory mandate for licensed social workers to obtain continuing education (CE) credits went into effect. Until then, New York was the only state to not require CE for social workers (Schachter, 2014). The new law requires all licensed social workers (LCSWs and LMSWs) to obtain 36 CE contact hours over a 3-year registration period. Although the statute does not require new licensees to accumulate CE hours until after their first 3-year license registration period, it does apply to most of the 56,000 licensed social workers in New York State, and the 21,000 specifically in New York City (New York State Education Department, 2015c).

Mandates for social workers to engage in CE encodes in law a basic principle reflected in the National Association of Social Workers (NASW) *Standards for Continuing Professional Education.* As stated in the *Standards*, CE is "an essential activity for ensuring quality social work services for clients." The Standards point out that through CE, "new knowledge is acquired, skills are refined, professional attitudes are reinforced, and lives are changed" (NASW, 2003, p. 7).

This article examines the initial experience of the National Association of Social Workers New York City Chapter (NASW-NYC) in providing CE to licensed, MSW-level social workers, as well as the experience of licensed social workers who attended NASW-NYC's first conference, following the legal mandate going into effect, designed to provide CE credits. This article reviews what was involved in designing the conference, as well as the outcome, examined through the lens of a formative assessment.

Most important, evaluations that attendees completed are analyzed with the purpose of determining whether the intention of the NASW *Standards for Continuing Professional Education*—that the quality of social work services to clients be enhanced—was to some degree achieved. To comply with regulatory requirements of the State Education Department, in order to provide state-mandated CE, NASW-NYC developed a simple evaluation instrument (based on a 5-point Likert scale), which included whether the participants agreed that the offerings increased their knowledge of the subject matter and whether they expected to use what they had learned in their practice. Although the evaluation did not directly measure whether services were (or would be) enhanced, to the degree participants learned something new, and believed they would use it in their practice, can be viewed as an indicator of the potential for practice enhancement.

We first explore the impact of a statutory CE requirement by briefly comparing participation in NASW-NYC's CE programs before, and after, the law went into effect. The question being addressed is whether social workers were already engaged in CE, without the inducement provided by a legal mandate, or whether the necessity of participating in continuing education, to ensure licensure renewal, changed professional behavior.

Comparison of Participation Before and After the Mandate

Although New York State did not require social workers to engage in CE until 2015, NASW-NYC had launched its CE program in 1998, which continued through the fall of 2013. The program then resumed in 2015 when the new requirement went into effect. Prior educational offerings typically consisted of 3-hour and 6-hour workshops on a wide range of topics, from clinical practice to administration. Twelve to 15 workshops previously had been offered each year.

Workshops that addressed clinical practice were overwhelmingly better attended than those on other topics, such as administration. Ones that featured well-known professors of clinical practice tended to attract the most attendees and would quickly reach the maximum attendance of 50 participants, the limited capacity of the NASW-NYC meeting room. This response, however, was the exception and not the rule, with individual workshop attendance generally slightly above or below 20 participants. With regard to the topic of administration, attempts to provide experts on such subjects as grant development, moving from clinician to supervisor, and agency leadership never achieved capacity, with attendance below 20 being the norm.

An exception to the level of attendance in the workshops just noted occurred 1 year prior to the CE mandate going into effect when the new *Diagnostic and Statistical Manual of Mental Disorders* (5th ed.) (American Psychiatric Association, 2013) was being introduced, reflecting a range of new diagnostic classifications and other significant changes from previous editions (American Psychiatric Association, 2013). The demand among social workers was such that, after 140 registered for a workshop on this topic, a second one was held with a similar number of attendees.

Even though these workshops were not requisite at the time for CE credit, there was a feeling among many mental health professionals that understanding the new *Diagnostic and Statistical Manual of Mental Disorders* would become essential for complying with requirements for providing diagnoses, especially when third-party reimbursement would be involved. The belief that it was crucial for practitioners to comply with the new diagnostic requirements compelled many social workers to enroll, and attendance reflected this factor.

By comparison, once the mandate went into effect, workshops on similar topics (to those that had been previously available) reached our maximum meeting space capacity in every instance, and for several offerings the interest was great enough to warrant renting a larger space. For example, a 2015 workshop on cognitive behavioral therapy was attended by 194 social workers. Although this topic was popular prior to the new mandate going into effect, previously it had not attracted more than 50 attendees.

Another indication of the surge in participation in CE offerings was an outcome of timing. The registration for NASW-NYC's 1-day conference commenced just 3 months after the law went into effect. Although the leadership of NASW-NYC anticipated that there would therefore likely be a high demand to attend the conference (and obtained a space to accommodate more than 900 attendees), it was a surprise that registration reached capacity just 10 days after it was opened. The chapter had engaged in widespread marketing of the conference, given the possibility that attendance would not achieve the capacity permitted by the space, but it was not expected that the interest in attending would be so great that registration would have to be closed as quickly as it was. It is a reasonable assumption that the incipient legal requirement related to maintaining one's license, and therefore the ability to continue to practice, generated a totally new level of interest in signing up for CE offerings.

Designing the Conference and Selection of Educational Offerings

NASW-NYC's leadership, through a series of discussions prior to the CE law going into effect, made several decisions that determined what educational offerings would be available to licensed social workers who might choose to register for the conference. Therefore, focusing on the choices made in the conference design, and how the offerings were determined, is central to understanding the outcome of the conference and the experience of the social workers who participated.

Potential decisions included (a) deciding on the size of the conference, (b) determining how to base the conference on prior experience of the organization, (c) selecting what particular niche of potential offerings would be appropriate for NASW-NYC, and (d) choosing how both topics and presenters would be selected.

The role of the Continuing Education Planning Committee was pivotal in determining what the selections would be among these potential choices. However, prior to the formation of the planning committee, the officers of the NASW-NYC Board of Directors, facing the likelihood that a large portion of New York City's 21,000 licensed social workers would be looking for opportunities to participate in CE as soon as the mandate went into effect, decided to hold as large a 1-day conference as would be possible. Although this decision was based on a desire to become known for offering quality and responsive CE, for the future, as well as the present, this decision also was made out of a sense of responsibility and the realization that it might be difficult for many social workers to gain access to educational offerings while the new law was just going into effect. Hence, a venue for the conference was obtained that could accommodate more than 900 participants, with enough space for plenary sessions, and adequate rooms for breakout workshops.

The Planning Committee was comprised of social work leaders in NASW-NYC, many holding elected position on the Board of Directors, along with others who had previously served on the Board. The Committee members included experienced clinicians, educators, organizers, and administrators, representing both the public and nonprofit human service sectors, and evinced diversity in terms of race and gender.

Of particular importance to the members of this Committee was the choice of educational offerings. It was agreed that they should reflect (a) the impact of changing policies on practice, (b) new approaches to clinical and direct practice, and (c) the impact of current policies and trends on clients and their communities, including an examination of the selections through a social justice and racial equity lens.

Once the Planning Committee had decided on the broad categories to include in the conference, a call for proposals was drafted and sent out to the NASW-NYC membership, as well as to faculty at schools of social work in New York City and surrounding counties. Seventy-two proposals were received and reviewed by the Committee over the course of two 3-hour meetings. From the 72 proposals, 24 workshops were authorized. In addition, the Committee both determined the focus and selected the speakers for two plenary sessions that all conference participants would attend. The topics for these sessions were on national trends affecting oppressed communities in New York City and on the social determinants of health.

Conference Outcomes, Evaluations, and Experience of the Participants

Subsequently, on the day of the conference, these two plenary sessions and 24 workshops were held and attended by approximately 800 social workers, plus an additional 100 presenters and volunteers.

NASW-NYC, in compliance with regulatory requirements, conducted an evaluation of the plenary sessions and workshops. Like the instructors and the workshops themselves, the evaluation instrument (preapproved by the State Office of the Professions) was designed to elicit responses along a 5-point Likert scale on which respondents could rank the degree to which they agreed or disagreed with 12 statements, where 1 signified strong disagreement with the statement and 5 signified strong agreement. Statements addressed satisfaction with a speaker's expertise and communication ability, as well as whether attendees felt that the objectives for the educational offering were met. Other items solicited a response to such variables as the accessibility of the building and the convenience of the conference location.

In reviewing the evaluations, two items were of particular interest: "The content increased my knowledge of the subject matter" and "I will use this learning in my practice in the future." Arguably, these two questions may have the most direct bearing for shedding light on whether the goals of CE, as identified in the NASW (2003) *Standards for Continuing Professional Education*, were met as a result of attending the conference. According to these Standards, continuing education is about ensuring quality social work services for clients. It is expected that, through CE, participants will acquire new knowledge and their skills will be increased (NASW, 2003). Although no contemporary evaluations can reveal whether client services will be enhanced, responses to these two items may be considered indicators of whether the conference offerings were perceived by participants to have potential impact on their knowledge, skills, and practice.

A total of 649 conference participants (76%) completed the evaluations electronically (approximately two to three weeks after the conference), addressing each of the four educational offerings (two plenary sessions and two workshops) that all participants were able to attend. Composite scores for 23 offerings were examined: two plenary sessions and 21 workshops. (It is noted that evaluations for three of the 24 workshops, representing perhaps up to 10% of attendees, were not available.)

To aid in the comparisons among the several statements, all scores of 4.0 or higher were considered to reflect a greater degree of agreement with the individual statements, whereas scores below 4.0 were considered to reflect less agreement with the statement. Although this cutoff point is arbitrary, it does permit differences to emerge, even if small. It is noted overall, however, that the differences among some of the scores reported here range from 4.6 on the high end to 3.1 on the low end. Although tests of significance were not performed, it is reasonable to assume that such differences reflect the actual experience of participants and therefore are useful to examine.

For the item, "The content increased my knowledge of the subject matter," there were ratings of 4.0 or higher for 15 of the 23 educational offerings, or 65%. Of these, 39% ($n = 9$) of them were rated between 4.1 and 4.4. Two offerings were scored at or above 4.5, and four rated at 4.0. There were ratings below 4.0 for 35% of the workshops ($n = 8$). Of these, 22% ($n = 5$) were between 3.6 and 3.9, and 13% ($n = 3$) were below 3.5.

For the item, "I will use this learning in my practice in the future," there were ratings of 4.0 for 13 educational offerings, or 57%. Of these, 35% ($n = 8$) scored between 4.1 and 4.4. One workshop was rated at or above 4.5, and four were rated at 4.0. Ten workshops scored below 4.0, representing 43% of the offerings. Four were between 3.6 and 3.9, and six were at 3.5 or slightly lower.

As previously mentioned, the NASW-NYC Continuing Education Planning Committee was especially interested in providing educational options in the areas of (a) the impact of changing policies on practice, (b) approaches to clinical and direct practice, and (c) the implications of current trends for clients, and the communities they came from—with an examination of each of these through considerations of social justice and racial equity. Table 1 reflects these three categories of workshops, as well as one offering on program evaluation and planning. The table lists the educational offerings that fall under each category and provides the ratings for each of the statements that were being considered.

Five of the 23 workshops were classified as reflecting policy impacting practice. The overall composite score for these five was rated by participants as 3.7 in relation to increasing their knowledge and 3.6 for the likelihood that the information from the offering would be used in the future.

Eleven workshops were identified as falling under the classification of new developments in clinical or direct practice. Overall, participants in these workshops rated both variables (reflecting increased knowledge and the likelihood of using the information in the future) as 4.1.

Six educational offerings, including the two plenary sessions, were perceived as falling under the classification of "impact of current trends on communities." Those attending these sessions rated increased knowledge at 4.1 and the likelihood that the information would be utilized in the future at 3.9.

It is noted that, despite an interest in having educational offerings for administrators, only one workshop in this category, for program evaluation and planning, was held. (It also was the only one on the topic that had been submitted.) If supervision were to be included with administration, then one could conceptualize that three were held, but supervision was grouped with the offerings related to clinical and direct practice. This one workshop in the arena of administration was rated as 3.8 for increased knowledge and 3.5 for likelihood that the information would be used in the future.

Table 1. Evaluation Scores for 23 Educational Offerings by Topic Regarding "Whether Knowledge Was Increased" and "Learning Will Be Used in the Future."

	Increased knowledge	Will use in future
Educational offerings by type of topic		
• New policies impacting practice		
1. Behavioral Health Integration	4.0	3.8
2. Issues in Health Care	3.2	3.1
3. Trends in Aging	3.6	3.5
4. Transition to Medicaid Managed Care	4.1	4.0
5. Trends in Child Welfare	3.4	3.4
Composite score	3.7	3.6
• Developments in clinical and direct practice		
1. Culturally Competent Domestic Violence Intervention	4.4	4.2
2. Role of the Supervisor	3.5	3.5
3. Reflective Supervision Across Race, Diversity, and Intersectionality	4.6	4.6
4. Transgender Practice	4.5	4.3
5. HIV Prevention	3.6	3.4
6. When Trauma Does Not Stop	4.0	4.0
7. Adolescent Mental Health	4.0	4.0
8. Getting Unstuck: Navigating Impasses	4.1	4.0
9. Sand Tray Therapy for Childhood Trauma	4.4	4.4
10. End-of-Life Care	4.2	4.2
11. Ethics and Risk Management	4.2	4.2
Composite score	4.1	4.1
• Impact of trends on communities		
1. Social Determinants of Health [plenary session]	4.2	4.0
2. Social Work and Mass Incarceration	3.9	3.7
3. Immigration in NYC	4.0	3.7
4. Retooling Mental Health Models for Racial Relevance	3.6	3.7
5. Community Loss Indexes	4.4	4.4
6. National Trends Influencing Communities in NYC [plenary session]		4.3
Composite score	4.1	3.9
• Program evaluation and planning		
1. What the Data Tells Us	3.8	3.5

Note. Data were recorded on a Likert scale of 1 to 5, reflecting agreement with statements, where 1 signifies strong disagreement and 5 signifies strong agreement.

Discussion of the Findings: What the NASW-NYC Experience Tells US

The advent of the mandate in January 2015, that licensed social workers in New York acquire CE credits, immediately set in motion practitioner efforts to comply with the law. Although many social workers had voluntarily engaged in CE activities in the past, the new requirement had a major impetus on social workers seeking CE options.

An appropriate question is, What will be the benefits for licensed social workers, and through them, for the clients that they serve, by virtue of the now requisite hours of CE? Overall, it would seem fair to conclude from the data in Table 1 that participants in the NASW-NYC conference found value in the educational opportunity. The evaluations suggest that, for the majority of the educational offerings, knowledge of the subject matter increased and that there was perceived to be a likelihood of participants using the newly acquired knowledge and skills in their practice. Even for the workshops that were rated somewhat lower, all were in a positive direction, even if not as strong as might be desired.

It is important to remember that the NASW-NYC's Continuing Education Planning Committee was committed to providing educational options that addressed the impact of current trends on communities in which many of their clients reside. Underlying this Committee priority was the assumption that practitioners need to be equipped to understand and address the factors impinging on the lives of their clients, including poverty, mass incarceration, and racism. This presumption is connected to the high proportion of social work clients in New York City being persons of color, having low income, and facing a range of challenges that represent systemic societal oppression. However, it also was understood that many social workers prefer to attend educational offerings that will enhance their clinical practice, and in the past (prior to the CE mandate) attendees at NASW-NYC sessions tended to choose such workshops over other types of offerings.

The evaluations show that of the 11 offerings addressing clinical and direct practice and the six addressing issues affecting the community, participants were just about equal in "their knowledge being increased," but the "likelihood of using the information in one's practice" was slightly higher for the practice oriented sessions, although not by much.

Although the workshops on trends impacting communities and direct practice were rated in a very similar manner, such was not the case for the offerings that addressed the impact of policy on practice. They generally were rated lower in knowledge learned and in the likelihood of using the information in practice. This finding was surprising, given the assumption that understanding policies, especially related to behavioral managed care, and health care under the new Affordable Care Act, were undergoing major change. It was presumed that important and evolving knowledge of these developments was likely limited to executives and program directors, and that even they were unsure how the new policies would impact service delivery, given that the rules and regulations were still being refined. Our supposition that practitioners and supervisors might be curious about these emerging policies (and the likely impact on their practice) did not prevail.

To understand this outcome, one could question whether social workers attending these sessions already had this information, contrary to what was assumed. Other possibilities include (a) that many social workers are simply not that interested in addressing policy and (b) the presenters were not perceived as adequate to the task. The latter conclusion would appear to be unlikely. Data from the evaluations regarding the knowledge of the presenters, specifically for the policy-related workshops, show ratings that were relatively high. In other words, it does not appear that the workshops were rated somewhat lower due to disappointment with the presenters.

The Future of Continuing Education in New York City and Issues Needing Consideration

With the CE mandate now in effect, it is clear that the need for provision of quality educational offerings is just beginning. This article, by examining the early experience of NASW-NYC via its responsive conference (along with the evaluations by the social workers who attended), points to a range of issues that should be considered moving forward.

Perhaps the first one is the nature of the demand and the current availability of offerings. The New York State Office of the Professions requires a rigorous application to be completed in order to be approved as a provider of CE, and many potential providers may need time to learn the process and then to complete the application. When NASW-NYC first received approval from the Office of the Professions to be an authorized CE provider, it was number 27 in the state to receive such approval. Approximately one year later, there were more than 200 approved providers, and it is expected that this number will grow, perhaps substantially (New York State Education Department, 2015a).

The implication is that licensed social workers will have increasing choices as to where to obtain their credits and that it is not certain that the attendance at a conference such as held by NASW-NYC will continue to attract the large number of social workers that it did the 1st year of the implementation of the requirement.

On the other hand, the number of licensed social workers in New York City alone is so large, at 21,000, that demand for CE offerings will likely be quite strong. In effect, with a requirement for each licensee to acquire an average of 12 CE hours each year in order to accumulate 36 CE contact hours over 3 years, the total in New York City alone could amount to the need for an aggregate accumulation of 252,000 hours of CE in every year, give or take. In the context of this level of need, it is possible that an organization such as NASW-NYC will continue to be sought out by large numbers of licensees.

A second issue relates to the *type* of CE offerings that licensed social workers will choose. The CE regulations in New York provide for a list of acceptable subjects that are broad and nonspecific, allowing license holders a great deal of latitude, so long as the topic directly relates to enhancing social work practice and client well-being (New York State Education Department, 2015b). (Although some states have requirements for selected subjects, such as in ethics, New York State does not require specific subjects at this time.) For the NASW-NYC Continuing Education Planning Committee, a choice was made to emphasize the impact of trends on communities in which most social work clients reside, along with the prospective effect of emerging public policies on practice. NASW's niche specifically related to the theme of "Social Work in the City," and the need for practitioners to view their work through both an intersectionality and racial equity lens. It is an open question as to whether social workers will be attracted to such offerings in the future, should there be many other approved CE options to choose from; however, the NASW-NYC conference experience suggests that, at least for trends impacting client communities, there is considerable workshop interest. Whether social workers will choose to attend CE offerings related to policy, on the other hand, needs further exploration.

Finally, the question regarding whether CE offerings will enhance knowledge and strengthen practice, to benefit services to clients, must remain a focal issue. Evaluations that are typically used rely on participant self-reports (such as reflected here), which are valuable; but more rigorous approaches and summative assessments are needed to determine whether client well-being is enhanced as a result of social workers' now mandatory participation in CE. The whole point of CE rests on achieving this goal. In the meantime, measures that serve as indicators that practice is enhanced, and thereby likely to benefit clients, will continue to be an important focus of the overall CE program of NASW in New York City.

References

American Psychiatric Association. (2013). *Diagnostic and statistical manual of mental disorders* (5th ed.). Arlington, VA: Author.

National Association of Social Workers. (2003). *Standards for continuing professional education.* Washington, DC: Author.

New York State Education Department, Office of the Professions. (2015a). *Continuing education: Department approved providers.* Retrieved from http://www.op.nysed.gov/prof/sw/swceproviderlist.htm

New York State Education Department, Office of the Professions. (2015b). *Continuing education for licensed master social workers or licensed clinical social workers.* Retrieved from http://www.op.nysed.gov/prof/sw/part74.htm#sce

New York State Education Department, Office of the Professions. (2015c). *License statistics.* Retrieved from http://www.op.nysed.gov/prof/sw/swcounts.htm

Schachter, R. (2014). *New York expected to mandate continuing education in 2015.* National Association of Social Workers, New York City Chapter. Retrieved from http://www.naswnyc.org/?447

Continuing Education for the Emerging Social Work Profession in China: The Experiment in Shenzhen

Ching Man Lam, Miu Chung Yan, and Yan Liang

ABSTRACT

In-service training as a form of continuing professional education (CPE) is important for social work professionals to maintain their skills and enhance their knowledge for publicly accountable practice. These goals are concerns in Mainland China, which has experienced rapid development in social work since economic reforms started in the early 1980s. This article reports the findings of a qualitative study that explored the in-service training experience of 36 social workers in the major city of Shenzhen, an "important role model" for social work development in China. The findings reveal that participants expect in-service training to be practical and applicable, and their narrative accounts reveal first a disconnect between their needs and the in-service training provided, and second their quest for value-based training to sustain their commitment to the social work profession. To strengthen CPE for social workers in China, a more consultative, flexible, and customized approach, as well as an experiential learning model, are needed. In light of these findings, the authors discuss the role and functions of CPE in a China-specific context and reflect on how CPE can be better delivered to meet the needs of current social workers in China.

Introduction

Becoming a competent social worker requires a commitment to an ongoing learning process. In many countries, formal social work training is a basic qualification to become a member of the social work profession. Although systematic learning processes in classrooms and in field placement can equip social work students with values, skills, and knowledge, formal social work training at university or professional school level alone cannot always fully prepare students to handle clients' complex needs and situations. Thus, new staff at social service organizations often are expected to pick up both codified knowledge, contained in policies and manuals, and cultural knowledge, such as habitual ways of doing business (Eraut, 2010), through systematic induction programs.

However, these induction programs are necessary but not sufficient. Given constantly changing social problems and social needs, competent social workers need to engage regularly in self-improvement, namely, updating knowledge and upgrading skills through in-service training. In a nutshell, the purpose of such continuous training is to help social workers renew and update their expertise in order to enhance their performance (Turcotte, Lamonde, & Beaudoin, 2009). As Clarke (2001) noted, in-service training is a means to assure accountability in the profession, which is funded largely by public money and seeks to achieve public policy goals. The prevailing ideology of evidence-based practice also requires social workers to constantly learn and employ new techniques in their practice in order to provide appropriate and high-quality service (Barfoed & Jacobsson, 2012).

Indeed, in many countries that have a social work licensing system, in-service training is organized as continuing professional education (CPE), a mandatory licensure renewal requirement imposed on its members as a means of ensuring accountability and high-quality service provision.

CPE and Social Work in China

Social work in China has experienced rapid development over the last three decades. Chinese society, while enjoying the fruits of reform, is experiencing increasing social demands from its citizens—caused by both mounting social problems and the worsening wealth gap, on one hand, and a desire to improve the quality of life and a growing consciousness of human and citizen rights, on the other (Leung, Yip, Huang, & Wu, 2012).

The government has undertaken a series of actions in response to these demands, seeking to maintain social stability toward the larger goal of building "a harmonious society" (Wang & Yuan-Tsang, 2009). A principal target has been to restructure and modernize the existing social service system, which had relied mainly on volunteers. The system has been rearranged and is now made up of work units (*Danwei*, which refers to state-owned enterprises and public institutions); community residents' organizations; local service units of the Ministry of Civil Affairs; and a few semi-governmental or government-supported non-government organizations such as the All-China Women's Federation, Communist Youth League of China, and All-China Federation of Trade Unions. The operational mechanism is that the government branches are responsible for financial input, support of social services, and policy planning and implementation, whereas the sem-igovernmental organizations will provide direct services in their own sector for specific client cohorts, such as youth, women, and workers.

In addition to this restructuring, the government also has focused on modernization via two major interrelated measures. The first measure involved the reintroduction of professional social work training to the tertiary education system (i.e., the universities and vocational colleges in mainland China). This move began as early as 1988 (Yan & Tsang, 2005). However, the formal development of social work education remained slow until the mid-2000s, when the central government committed to an immense investment in expanding social welfare services, including a plan to increase the number of social workers to 1.45 million by 2020 (Gao & Yan, 2014). As a result, the number of social work training institutions (and social work practitioners) has recently witnessed significant growth. By the end of 2014, the number of schools offering social work degree programs reached 310, with around 30,000 graduates annually, and with 104 higher-education institutes offering postgraduate training in social work as well (Jiang, 2015).

The second measure involved the establishment of the social service system. Under the economic reform, the work units have been released from their social welfare and service responsibilities. Instead, a new entity, social work service organizations (SWSO), gradually has been established (Gao & Yan, 2014). According to the Ministry of Civil Affairs (2014), which oversees these developments, the 2015 budget included 200 million Renminbi (approximately US$30 million) to support social organizations in delivering social assistance, social welfare programs, community service projects, and professional social work services. Consequently the social service sector has flourished, especially in the coastal regions and developed cities. In 2014, there were 3,522 social service organizations nationwide, with Guangdong Province topping the list at 770 (Jiang, 2015). Still, with this promising expansion of professional social work service, the shortcomings of social work education became clear and significant.

In the early 2000s, the Ministry of Education standardized the curriculum of social work programs, which is largely based on a generalist model. Students are taught social work history, values and principles, practice methods (mainly case, group, and community), policy, and research (Yan & Tsang, 2005). Nonetheless, as the literature (e.g., Yan, Gao, & Lam, 2013; Yan, Ge, Cheng, & Tsang, 2009) has shown, although most social work programs in China do include courses that focus on practical knowledge and skills training, most of these courses remain at the theoretical level. The lack of qualified teachers and field educators hinders the quality of skills training, especially in terms of the competence and readiness of social work graduates to enter the field. Owing to these current shortcomings, China's new social work graduates are, to a large extent, unprepared for direct practice in the field and hence for meeting the needs of clients they serve (Lam & Yan, 2015; Yan et al., 2013). Meanwhile, most government service units, and the newly established social work service organizations, also lack trained personnel who can provide proper practicum training and ongoing professional supervision to these newly graduated social workers. The current induction programs— usually in the form of prejob training covering orientation to the agency, briefing on administrative procedures, basic social work knowledge, and skills—greatly lag behind the new workers' needs (Yan et al., 2013).

In view of these inadequacies, in Shenzhen, a major city of approximately 10 million people known for its ambitious development of social work services (Chan, Ip, & Lau, 2009), a systematic and government-led CPE program has been piloted as a possible solution to meet the training needs of this now rapidly growing team of service providers. But so far, to the best of our knowledge, no one has studied how (and how well) this experiment in Shenzhen—or in-service professional training in China, generally—works. In this article we address the topics of the impact of CPE on social workers in China, the kinds of in-service training social workers find useful and effective, and ways to better design and provide CPE to accommodate different emerging needs. The authors also attempt to provide answers to these questions, based on the findings of a qualitative study of a group of social workers specifically in Shenzhen.

Social Work Development in Shenzhen

Shenzhen has been an important role model for social work development in China (Lam & Yan, 2015), particularly after the local government issued several milestone documents in 2007 that laid down the framework for the city's social work manpower and social welfare services. Indeed, the local government, especially the Civil Affairs Bureau, has played a crucial function in boosting the development of social work, providing endorsement, financial support, and policy frameworks. Most important, it took the initiative to integrate and embed social work in the existing social service infrastructure. Shenzhen was one of the first cities in China to pilot SWSOs, and today it has 122 (Du, 2015).

In addition, social work development in Shenzhen has long been influenced by the social work profession in Hong Kong because of its geographical proximity. Since 2008, professional supervisors have been brought from Hong Kong to oversee and to support social work practitioners hired by the SWSO, which is a distinguishing feature of Shenzhen-based social work (Hung, Ng, & Fung, 2010). However, hiring supervisors from Hong Kong is expensive, and due to budget limitations, as well as to the increased number of locally trained supervisors, this cross-border supervision has been gradually phased out. The removal of Hong Kong supervision now poses challenges to local social work practitioners and service organizations in terms of maintaining service quality (Lam & Yan, 2015). Unfortunately, the SWSO still lack the professional and financial capacity to ensure the performance of their social workers. To address this situation, a more economical and sustainable approach is needed.

The Shenzhen Association of Social Workers (SZASW) has been assigned the key role of providing in-service training, in the form of CPE, for all social workers working in Shenzhen. SZASW, which is the government-operated umbrella organization of social work practitioners and social service organizations, has a fourfold mandate: to serve as a link between social workers and the government, to manage the city's registered social workers, to coordinate and administer professional supervision, and to regulate professional standards. Thus, it has a strong interest in ensuring the competency of Shenzhen's cadre of registered social workers.

In response to two national policy papers—"The Opinions on Strengthening the Construction of Social Work Professional Personnel" and "The Medium- and Long-Term Talent Development Plan of Social Work Professional Personnel (2010–2020)"—issued by the central government, SZASW passed "The Implementation of Regulations of Social Work Professionals' Continuing Professional Education in Shenzhen" (hereafter "the Regulations"), which took effect on December 10, 2010. This document set up trial CPE requirements for social workers in Shenzhen, and after two amendments were made, the Regulations became permanent in December 2014.

The Current Shenzhen system has two tiers of social workers. The first tier is registered social workers (*Shehuigongzuozhe*), who have passed the national accreditation examination but do not necessarily have social work training. Experienced social workers from this tier can be promoted to junior supervisor or supervisor. The other tier is registered social welfare workers (*Shehuigongzuoyuan*), who are mainly nontrained social workers with practical training of not less than 5 days, plus attaining a target score set by SZASW in the national career accreditation examination.

According to the Regulations, all social workers employed in Shenzhen must attend CPE training. A minimum of 120 learning hours (45 minutes per learning hour) of continuing education every year is required for registered social workers, whereas 80 hours is required for registered social welfare workers. (Among these 120 learning hours, at least 8 hours must relate to professional values and ethics.) CPE credits can be earned in many ways, and training can be in various formats, including attending seminars and conferences, participating in various formal visits, taking online courses or attending formal social work classes, or publishing in academic journals (Shenzhen Association of Social Workers, 2014). CPE activities and programs are mainly organized and delivered by SZASW. SWSO (and other training agencies accredited by SZASW) also provide some CPE courses, which must be assessed and reviewed by an expert panel at SZASW to assure acknowledgment of CPE hours. In spite of this, the content of training courses varies; some are quite "therapeutic" in nature, as quite a number of the trainers have a psychology background. For example, analytical psychological tools frequently are taught, but participants reflected that frequently only the concepts are introduced. With scant opportunity to do therapeutic work, as well as a weak mastering of the techniques, attendees perceived the training as impractical. At the other extreme, some training courses are very general, covering broad principles, or simply arranging visits to local or Hong Kong agencies.

Methodology

The study was conducted under the ethical protocols approved by the Chinese University of Hong Kong. Qualitative in-depth individual interviews were conducted with 36 social workers in Shenzhen, China. Using a purposive sampling method, the researchers identified and obtained access to settings where information-rich individuals were available to provide details about their personal experiences and perceptions (Patton, 1990). Access to these individuals was made possible by support from SZASW and the Hong Kong Institute of Social Service Development, a Hong Kong–based organization that provides supervision to social workers in Shenzhen. An invitation letter, with information on the purpose of this study, including its interview procedures and the selection criteria, was sent to each potential participant. The inclusion criteria for sampling were social workers who (a) had formal training in social work, (b) held social work positions in Shenzhen at the time of their interviews, and (c) would provide consent to be interviewed.

Thirty-six participants (8 male and 28 female social workers) took part in this study. Their ages ranged from 23 to 30 ($M = 25.6$), with work experience of 3 months to 3.5 years ($M = 17.5$ months). They were working in a variety of service settings—eight participants in youth and school services, nine in child and family services, 14 in community-based programs, three in health and drug programs, one in mediation service, and one with migrant laborers. Participants came from 13 agencies and were graduates of the social work programs of 26 universities in China. Regarding education level, three had postgraduate qualifications and 33 had undergraduate degrees.

Individual face-to-face interviews were conducted by either the first author or her research assistant, an MSW student at the Chinese University of Hong Kong. Interviews followed a semi-structured interviewing guide and explored the participants' working experiences, perceived training needs, experiences with in-service training, and reflections on their in-service trainings. All interviews were tape-recorded and fully transcribed (in Chinese) by student helpers. The transcripts were analyzed with the assistance of NVivo 10, a qualitative data analysis computerized software package. A thematic approach was used to analyze the data. Transcripts first were coded, and all codes then were categorized and recategorized until mutually exclusive themes were identified. To ensure validity of the subsequent findings, participants were invited to a focus group to discuss the preliminary findings. The focus group was held in Shenzhen and facilitated by the three authors.

Feedback collected from these focus groups positively validated the analysis. (Only quotations we cited anonymously in the following section were translated into English, and back-translation was used to ensure accuracy. Pseudonyms were assigned to respondents in alphabetical order and according to gender.)

Findings

Based on the 36 participants' experiences, observations, and perceptions related to in-service training, three themes were identified: (a) an emphasis on practicality and applicability, (b) a disconnect between in-service training and training needs, and (c) a quest for values-based training to sustain commitment.

Emphasis on Practicality and Applicability

The participants generally had positive comments regarding their continuing education. They perceived the trainings as helpful in improving and consolidating their knowledge and skills. The participants frequently used phrases like "*shi-jian*" (practical), "*shi-wu*" (matters related to actual practice), "*shi-yong*" (useful), "*shi-zai*" (substantial, not empty), "*shi-ji*" (realistic, applicable, feasible), and "*qie-shi*" (practicable, down-to-earth) as criteria for their evaluation of the effectiveness of the training. The Chinese character "实" (*shi*) strongly implies the concepts of practicability and applicability. Indeed, most of the participants expected in-service training to improve their actual practice. Ana, a social worker with 1.5 years of experience who worked as a frontline worker at a family service center, shared this view:

> I don't think induction training was useful. I found in-service training more effective than induction training because, after having some practical experience, then going for in-service training, it gave us more opportunity to integrate theory and practice. In terms of operation, [in-service training] is like a reminder of how to practice in the future. ... It is like we tried and then we know. ... I think actual practice should come first, and then integration with theories that we have learned. Because in school, what we largely learned was about theories but with no practice. After we have practice, we can integrate the theories. I think this kind of integration is better.

According to Ana, in-service training helped her integrate theory with her actual experience. Ana also pointed out that in their undergraduate studies, she and her fellow social work students were not trained well enough to become practicing social workers. The lack of practical training was particularly challenging to the participants who were new graduates. Many of them felt strongly that in-service training should not be about abstract theories and philosophies; instead, they longed for practical ways of doing social work. As Betty, a frontline social worker who had graduated 2 years earlier, said,

> I prefer those in-service trainings where the speakers talk more about things related to practice. People like us, university graduates with little experience, are quite inadequate in practice. So, don't talk about theories or grand ideas, or that sort of stuff. Tell us more about practice.

The format of in-service training matters; lectures in big groups are not preferred. As Cathy, a junior supervisor with 2 years of practice, said, "If the scale of the in-service training activity is too big, it becomes a formality and too general." Therefore, many participants remarked that to help them with theory and practice integration, experiential learning is a more helpful and impactful form of in-service training. They therefore preferred training that involved simulation exercises and immediate feedback, which made them (particularly the new graduates) feel more "*ta-shi*" (assured and confident) when practicing in the field.

> I feel that probably in-service training with a participatory element is more useful. If only talking, particularly reading directly from the texts, (Interviewer: It is not useful?) Yes. If possible, if I have more opportunities to participate, I will feel more confident. No matter how. — Dorothy (a junior supervisor in a community service setting with 5 years of experience).

Dorothy's perspective was shared by another junior supervisor, Eva (with 3 years of experience in a drug-abuse setting), who recalled one episode at an in-service training:

> He [the trainer] trained us how to lead activities. Then he gave us experience by asking us to run groups. In the process, we shared some ideas: why he used this approach to run the group, what were the theories behind it, and how we felt in the process. It was direct experience ... just like that. With more participation, the learning is deeper.

The participants' eagerness to learn practical skills through in-service training also was reflected in their preference for a certain kind of trainer. Those with actual field experience were much preferred by the participants, as these trainers were more likely to have personally experienced similar difficulties and struggles. For instance, according to Fred, a junior supervisor with 4 years of experience in a medical setting,

> The speakers, most of them have experienced the bitterness; they have the wisdom and experience. Once [I] interact with them, they know immediately what problems I have encountered in work. They have experience in how to resolve them [the problems]. If you really seriously listen, you will learn a lot from their experience, including knowledge and skills.

Comparatively speaking, to many participants, the social work scholars, particularly social work educators in China were not preferred because they were seen as lacking sufficient relevant experience in actual direct practice. As Gina, a supervisor with 5 years' experience working in the community-service field, commented,

I think the qualifications of the instructors are quite important. ... The instructors invited by SZASW can be classified into two major groups. One is scholars from mainland China who gave me a very official and very bureaucratic impression ... quite general and not getting to the point. They were educated in China, particularly in sociology, so to me, their stuff is cliché, nothing new. But the scholars from Hong Kong and Taiwan gave me an impression that they were very professional and respectful in their work. The training they provided gave me a genuine feeling of learning something useful ... because now we don't need those empty speeches. We need something that is more practical.

The participants' views clearly articulated ideas of practicability and applicability. A strong expectation of being equipped with practical and hand-on skills was apparent in the narratives of the research participants.

Disconnect Between In-Service Training and Training Needs

At present, SZASW plays multiple significant roles with respect to in-service training: provider, coordinator, and accreditor. A top-down approach has been used in planning and implementation of CPE in-service training. In other words, the programs are chosen and designed based on SZASW's assessments. Consultation with frontline social workers is minimal. Inevitably, this curriculum protocol causes a disconnect between the program and the needs of the trainees.

The training theme was decided by SZASW. Sometimes, they might ask for our perspective because, working here, we have experienced different and difficult situations. Some of us are quite confused. If they could ask for our opinion about the content of the training before they decide on the training theme, it would be better. — Helen (a social worker working in a women's rights setting, with 2 years of experience)

Like Helen, many participants suggested that the trainings should be more focused and targeted to their needs. To do so, their voices needed to be heard.

I feel that they should first understand the needs of frontline social workers. What kinds of knowledge do frontline social workers need? Which areas should be enhanced? In which areas are we inadequate? If they understand us more, and based the training on our needs, it would be more targeted. It will be easier for us to learn this stuff. — Kevin (a social worker with 2 years of experience in a youth service setting)

Meanwhile, without proper consultation, social workers often tend to become passive recipients. This reality is particularly problematic for those novices who do not always know their own needs. As a local supervisor pointed out,

There are quite a lot of trainings: different, diverse, and varied. However...social workers now are quite likely to not have a clear understanding of their own position. So, they may not be clear about what kind of training they may need, because I don't even know my own position...Since they themselves don't know about their needs, they are passive in training. Yes, in terms of social workers' training needs, maybe, some of them are very active, but as a whole, most of them are a bit passive. — Laura (a junior supervisor with 3 years of experience in a community-service setting)

Being a passive recipient may undermine the effects of training. Under the mandatory system, social workers often attend in-service training just for the sake of getting the requisite CPE credits to fulfill the registration renewal requirement. As a result, there is a risk that the mandatory nature of in-service training may render the trainees' participation a formality rather than an occasion for encouraging professional development.

I think the intention is good. [The training] aims to offer us ongoing learning. This is a continuing education process. However, I think that if your purpose is to arrange in-training activities to achieve a hard indicator—but those trainings are not useful, not fitting our needs as social workers, just forcing us to participate—then the effects will not be obvious. — Maria (a social worker with 2 years of experience in the labor rights field)

Many of us attend training just to finish a task, that is, to earn credits. If you don't have enough credits, you cannot complete your annual registration. I've noticed that many people attend in-service training activity but do not seriously or carefully listen. I think [they] do not benefit much." — Nancy (a social worker with 2 years of experience in a community-service setting)

Although the good intentions of SZASW are well understood by the participants, the current arrangement of in-service training provides little flexibility and often lacks responsiveness to the workers' actual needs. Some participants lamented that it was demanding and unrealistic to ask social workers to fulfill the 120-hour requirement. As Ana, a social worker with 15 years' experience at a family-service center, commented,

Too much — [SZASW] requires each person to have 120 credit hours. Our work at [X family center] actually is very busy. I have to run activities, plan and recruit. These tasks use a lot of my time. Each year, I still need to complete the credit hours, and I feel like I'm squeezing time from the gaps between my teeth to attend. I feel this will make us very tired. They just don't consider our needs.

In Shenzhen, under the service purchasing arrangement, some SWSO provide contractual services to government social service units by hiring social workers and then deploying them to these service settings. These outstationed workers face pressure not only from work but also from the service units, which expressed dissatisfaction when these workers needed to use their contracted service time for training. As Olga, a social worker stationed at the local judicial bureau, told us, "It is indeed very stressful for us to take so much time to attend training because where we are accountable is the service unit. Many service unit leaders think that we spend too much time on training." To resolve these problems, participants consistently suggested that better planning would be useful, based on a proper evaluation of the availability and expressed needs of the social workers.

> I feel that in-service training should be based on what we need or are interested in. They can conduct opinion surveys of us, and then based on the results of the survey they can arrange some [training]. That is, make an annual or quarterly in-service training plan. In this way, we could adjust our work and training. — Peter (a social worker with 3 months of experience in the youth services field)

The participants' views reveal discontent with the current top-down approach and a concern about their perceived disconnect between in-service training and participant training needs. Although they are the key stakeholder of in-service training, social workers have seldom been consulted or involved in the planning process. In turn, they frequently have become passive recipients.

The Quest for Values-Based Training to Sustain Commitment

Despite the fact that SZASW has offered in-service training on a variety of subjects and many participants have explicitly expressed the need for skill pursuit, many participants also enunciate the need for a reinforcement of social work values. To many, their commitment to and affinity toward social work values is what drove them to enter—and stay in—the profession. However, in Shenzhen there has been a high staff turnover in the social work field, partly due to low salaries and partly because of low job satisfaction. This high turnover rate may reflect a diminishing commitment to the social work profession. Indeed, many participants observed that, as time goes by, they and their colleagues experience a decrease in enthusiasm for and faith in social work. Very often, work becomes a routine struggle, and their commitment to social work values fades. Therefore, they hoped that some of the in-service training activities could inspire them by reminding them of their commitment to social work values. As Ray, a social worker with 8 months of experience in a community-service setting, said,

> In this way, it will be more useful, maybe, to provide more in-service training about social work values? Because social work needs to be value-based, right? For example, after working with service recipients for too long, gradually, [we] feel that many of our values are useless. Then we feel like we are working in a very routine way. Sometimes it feels like my values are fading.

Ray's tone and expression showed that he appreciated the value component of social work education and that he expected value-centered teaching would sustain social workers' commitments.

Sam, a junior social supervisor with 3 years of experience in a labor-rights setting, had a similar view on how to improve existing CPE training.

> It is more important to go deeper in the area of social work ethics, because we social workers in Shenzhen do not have a very high commitment to social work. A portion of social workers take social work only for a job, a source of income, or as a stepping stone to apply for civil-service or other jobs. If [in-service training] could further strengthen our social work ethics, it would be better.

Because the topics on social work values and ethics can be "rather boring" and "not attractive," as some participants commented, many suggested that training, particularly in the vague areas of values and ethics, should be experiential. As Dorothy, a supervisor with 2 years' experience in a community-service setting, said,

> Actually I think they [values] are very important. However, if, let's say, they [trainers or speakers] only list all these values [without discussion], it is not sufficient … but there is a way [of teaching], by pointing out some dilemmas in social work values that you have come across, which we can discuss. This gives us a deeper impression.

Several participants shared the view that trainers who are good at displaying their passion and commitment to social work values will be those who can be genuine and convincing, infusing the training with personal stories and reflections on ethical dilemmas. By talking about their own experiences, the speakers can shed more light on the actual meaning and implications of social work values and on the attitudes and viewpoints that reinforce their commitment to stay at their jobs and in the profession. As explained by Tina, a junior supervisor with 2 years of experience in a women's-rights setting,

> All three of [the trainers] talked about social work values. That is the most important thing in the service process. They gave me a feeling that the important element of this job is not about techniques or skills, or competence, or qualification. Skills are important, but the weight of these should not be that much. Instead, we need compassion, sensitivity, empathy, and passion. These things are more important in our work.

Tom, a social worker with 1 year of experience in a family-service setting, also shared his experience of a training session conducted by a social work educator from Hong Kong. He revealed how the trainer boosted his morale and widened his perspective.

> The training by [speaker's name] was quite touching. It changed my perspective. For example, he explicitly said one thing, that is, many social workers in the Shenzhen area have an expectation of striving for social equality and social justice. However, there are many [unequal] policies in Shenzhen. We are governed by these policies, so it is very difficult [to make a change]. He had a statement that is very touching: "It is very difficult, extremely difficult! But if it is not difficult, why do we need social workers?" This is what social work should do, it should be this way, right?

In sum, in-service training is not only about enhancing or updating the knowledge and skills of social workers. It has a very important career maintenance function for social work in Shenzhen, the development of which is still in an infancy stage. CPE is a crucial measure to ensure the commitment of social workers to stay in their jobs and in the profession.

Discussion

If CPE is to assure the self-enhancement and public accountability of the social work profession, then it is crucial for the rapidly increasing number of social workers in China. As a city that leads in the development of social work in China, Shenzhen's experience is unique but revealing. As noted, although social work education in China has exponentially expanded since 1988, unfortunately a majority of social work educators have never practiced social work themselves. Their teaching is largely theoretical, as reported both by participants of this study and in the literature. In addition, field education is still underdeveloped (Yan et al., 2013). A great majority of new graduates therefore lack practical experience and hence are not well prepared for practice. This reality is a major reason why, when the Shenzhen government first introduced social work to the city, they wisely imported supervisors from Hong Kong who were expected to help these new practitioners integrate theories that they had learned in school with actual practice in the field (Hung et al., 2010).

Consequently, the withdrawal of these Hong Kong social work supervisors left this problem unresolved. The high turnover rate of social workers in Shenzhen, as observed by our participants, also leads to the problem of the underprepared local supervisors not yet capable of taking over a supervisory role. Therefore, although the in-service training programs initiated and organized by SZASW are a reasonable move toward establishing a sustainable system—to ensure the accountability of the social work profession and to provide opportunities for members' own self-enhancement—to a certain extent, they also can be seen as an alternative and economical approach to filling in the gap in supervision. Learning from our participants, we were able to identify at least five issues that are critical in order for CPE to be successful in Shenzhen.

First, as reflected in our findings, the CPE system in Shenzhen is a government-driven initiative. Indeed, in the context of China, government has the most significant role in the making of social work (Gao & Yan, 2014). However, a centralized, top-down system, without proper consultation, may cause a disconnect between what in-service training offers and what social workers feel they actually need. Because China's social work development is still in the infancy phase, appropriate self-enhancement opportunities outside the government domain are very limited, and therefore it is understandable that the government will take the initiative to organize and deliver such training. Nonetheless, making government-driven in-service training work well is challenging, given that the actual needs of social workers vary due to diversity in their nature of work and the clientele served. As such, involving these professional adult learners in developing the objectives, content, and evaluation procedures should be a key future component in designing and delivering CPE. Meanwhile, different organizations have different codified and cultural knowledge that likely cannot be effectively transmitted through a common CPE approach. As our findings show, participants generally prefer a more flexible and decentralized approach, which can be better customized to their specific needs. Certainly they are asking for a more consultative approach, which would allow them the opportunity to voice their needs in the planning process.

Second, are 120 credit hours per year necessary for Shenzhen social workers? So far, there is no international minimum standard for CPE hours in social work. Moreover, although most countries have established a fixed annual number of requisite CPE credits, the ways to earn these credits are flexible and diverse. For instance, the Social Workers Registration Board in Hong Kong suggests 60 CPE hr per year on a voluntary basis for registered social workers to maintain their professional competency. In Canada, 40 CPE hours per year are required for ongoing renewal of registration. In England, the condition is 90 hours over 3 years. In the United States, from 12 to 48 CPE hours are expected, depending on each state's policies (Hong Kong Social Worker Registration Board, 2015). Nevertheless, regardless of the legal requirements of CPE for relicensure or recertification, in most cases, CPE credits can be earned in a variety of ways—formal training programs, short courses, internal agency training, online seminars, professional publication, self-study, volunteer work for community organizations, or via relaxation activities.

Comparatively speaking, the mandatory annual requirement of 120 credit hours for Shenzhen social workers may be excessive. As noted by many of our participants, this high threshold has put a burden on their already overloaded schedules. Thus, to a certain extent, CPE in Shenzhen has become a formality and a bureaucratic burden to many social workers. Attending in-service training is seen as being more focused on public accountability than on self-enhancement or professional development. It becomes simply an additional administrative requirement. As a result, the original intention of in-service training may be lost and goal displacement may occur.

That observation leads to the third concern: how to encourage the social workers to become self-motivated. The Shenzhen situation is that, although the choices of CPE courses on paper seem plentiful, social workers actually have few options for CPE, and most of the current approved trainings are theoretical in focus, rather than being centered on equipping them with new skills for work. In addition, CPE should be not only for performing specific tasks at work but also for fostering multidimensional personal and professional growth. With a broader and more integrative view of CPE, together with sufficient resources and support provided for social workers to pursue CPE training, participants will be more self-motivated and able to better benefit from the experience.

With regard to course format, most training courses have adopted the traditional educational model, with top-down professional–participant interaction, and with the goal to "educate" the social workers. According to Freire (1970), this traditional "banking" concept of education and training makes participants passive learners and gives them a feeling of inadequacy. To ensure successful CPE programs, responsive to learner needs, courses must be conducted with a more interactive format and with a greater focus on participants' self-development of reflective practice (Goldstein, 2001).

The fourth concern is about the goals of CPE in Shenzhen. It is widely agreed that CPE is a professional commitment and is essential for professional growth and development. The goal of CPE is to improve professional practice, avoid professional obsolescence, maintain currency of professional knowledge and skill, and ensure service quality so as to adapt to the changing world and shifting responsibilities (Cervero, 2001; Clarke, 2001; Faherty, 1979). However, considering the fact that social work education in China currently lacks practical components, and many social workers have not received formal training, CPE needs to supplement the still inadequate professional education and supervision in the workplace (Lam & Yan, 2015). This observation connects again to the question of whether 120 hours of CPE is needed for Shenzhen social workers. If CPE is used to supplement the inadequate present professional training and supervision, then one could argue perhaps that 120 hours may be reasonable, or not sufficient.

Last but not the least is the choice of trainers. The "people factor" (Lam, 2008) and the trainers' methods of facilitating the training process (Lam, 2011) are critical variables for effective CPE training. As reflected in the participants' narratives, the choice of instructors is the key. Taking the specific China situation into consideration, social work educators from mainland China may be a reasonable choice if training relates to policies or policy analysis. However, for skills training and facilitation of integration, trainers should have practical experience, be passionate about their work, and have optimistic attitudes toward people. These kinds of trainers will be able to teach by virtue of who they are and demonstrate their own experience. Learning from personal stories of experienced social workers can be inspirational.

Conclusion

In-service training as a form of CPE is important for social work professionals to maintain their self-enhancement for publicly accountable practice. This is particularly important for social work in China, which is still in its infancy. The example of Shenzhen, as reported in this article, indicates that in-service training has an important role to play, particularly when the formal curriculum and on-the-job supervision reflect deficiencies. Without a doubt, CPE plays a supplementary role to ensure quality of social work practice in China, and Shenzhen has provided a useful template. The way ahead will involve determining how to improve the quality of such training and make CPE better serve the needs of participants. What content is necessary for practicing social workers in China? What is the way forward now with the establishment of SZASW? Feedback from employers, trainers, and practitioners, along with independent research, is strongly suggested to improve the quality and relevance of CPE and in making the CPE curriculum responsive to the changing realities of practice.

Funding

Funding was provided by Direct Grant Research, CUHK SS11801.

References

Barfoed, E. M., & Jacobsson, K. (2012). Moving from "gut feeling" to "pure facts": Launching the ASI interview as part of in-service training for social workers. *Nordic Social Work Research, 2*(1), 5–20. doi:10.1080/2156857X.2012.667245

Cervero, R. M. (2001). Continuing professional education in transition: 1981–2000. *International Journal of Lifelong Education, 20*(1/2), 16–30.

Chan, T. K. T., Ip, D. F. K., & Lau, A. S. M. (2009). Social work professionalization in China: The case of Shenzhen. *China Journal of Social Work, 2*(2), 85–94. doi:10.1080/17525090902992222

Clarke, N. (2001). The impact of in-service training within social services. *British Journal of Social Work, 31*(5), 757–774. doi:10.1093/bjsw/31.5.757

Du, X. (2015, January 30). Shenzhen social workers jumped ship to Dongguan and Huizhou [Chinese]. *Nanfang Daily*. Retrieved from http://cpc.people.com.cn/BIG5/n/2015/0130/c87228-26476362.html

Eraut, M. (2010). Informal learning in the workplace. *Studies in Continuing Education, 26*(2), 247–273. doi:10.1080/158037042000225245

Faherty, V. (1979). Continuing social work education: Results of a Delphi survey. *Journal of Education for Social Work, 15*(1), 12–19. doi:10.1080/00220612.1979.10671539

Freire, P. (1970). *Pedagogy of the oppressed*, trans. Myra Bergman Ramos. New York: Continuum.

Gao, J. G., & Yan, M. C. (2014). Social work in making: The state and social work development in China. *International Journal of Social Welfare, 24*(1), 93–101. doi:10.1111/ijsw.12089

Goldstein, H. (2001). *Experiential learning: A foundation for social work education and practice*. Alexandria, VA: Council on Social Work Education.

Hong Kong Social Worker Registration Board (2015). Appendix 3: Reference of CPD requirements of professional and accreditation bodies. Retrieved from http://www.swrb. org.hk/cpd/en/CPD.asp?Uid=10

Hung, S. L., Ng, S. L., & Fung, K. K. (2010). Functions of social work supervision in Shenzhen: Insights from the cross-border supervision model. *International Social Work, 53*(3), 366–378. doi:10.1177/0020872809359864

Jiang, Y. (2015). 2014 National report on social work development. *SWChina Web*. Retrieved from http://news.swchina.org/industrynews/2015/0316/21002.shtml (in Chinese).

Lam, C. M. (2008). What makes a good program? A case study of a school admitting high academic achievers. *The Scientific World Journal: TSW Holistic Health & Medicine, 8*, 1027–1036. doi:10.1100/tsw.2008.123

Lam, C. M. (2011). Experiential and reflective learning approaches for the train-the-trainers program of Project P.A.T.H.S. *International Journal of Adolescence Medicine and Health, 23*(4), 305–310. doi:10.1515/IJAMH.2011.026

Lam, C. M., & Yan, M. C. (2015). Driving ducks onto a perch: The experience of locally trained Shenzhen supervisor. *China Journal of Social Work, 8*(2), 182–194. doi:10.1080/17525098.2015.1039169

Leung, T. T. F., Yip, N. M., Huang, R., & Wu, Y. (2012). Governmentality and the politicisation of social work in China. *British Journal of Social Work, 42*(6), 1039–1059. doi:10.1093/bjsw/bcs065

Ministry of Civil Affairs. (2014). *The Implementation Plan of Central Finance to Support Social Organizations in Participating in Social Service Projects in 2015*. Retrieved from http://big5. gov.cn/gate/big5/www.gov.cn/xinwen/2014-11/03/content_2774437.htm (in Chinese).

Patton, M. Q. (1990). *Qualitative evaluation and research methods* (2nd ed.). Newbury Park, CA: Sage.

Shenzhen Association of Social Workers. (2014). *The Implementation Regulations of Social Work Professionals' Continuing Professional Education in Shenzhen (Trial) (Amendment II)*. Retrieved from http://www.szswa.org/index/association/detail.jsp?id=24011 (in Chinese).

Turcotte, D., Lamonde, G., & Beaudoin, A. (2009). Evaluation of an in-service training program for child welfare practitioners. *Research on Social Work Practice, 19*(1), 31–41. doi:10.1177/1049731507313978

Wang, S., & Yuan-Tsang, A. (2009). The development of social work in China in the context of building a harmonious society [Chinese]. *China Social Sciences (Zhongguo Shehui Kexue), 5*, 128–140.

Yan, M. C., Gao, J. G., & Lam, C. M. (2013). The dawn is too distant: The experience of 28 social work graduates entering the social work field in China. *Social Work Education, 32*, 538–551. doi:10.1080/02615479.2012.688097

Yan, M. C., Ge, Z.-M., Cheng, S.-L., & Tsang, K. T. A. (2009). Imagining social work: A qualitative study of students' perspectives on social work in China. *Social Work Education, 28*, 528–543. doi:10.1080/02615470802368959

Yan, M. C., & Tsang, K. T. A. (2005). A snapshot on the development of social work education in China: A Delphi study. *Social Work Education, 24*(8), 883–901. doi:10.1080/02615470500342314

Continuing Education on Suicide Assessment and Crisis Intervention for Social Workers and Other Mental Health Professionals: A Follow-Up Study

Rebecca G. Mirick, Joanna Bridger, James McCauley, and Larry Berkowitz

ABSTRACT

Historically, graduate training programs have not taught suicide assessment and intervention skills in depth; therefore, the development of effective continuing education offerings is relevant and necessary for practicing social workers. Although the ability to increase knowledge and confidence is critical, a focus on competency-based education demands that training participants also incorporate the new skills into practice. This study evaluates a 6 hour continuing education program on suicide assessment and intervention. A one-group, pretest/posttest/3-month follow-up design assessed changes in knowledge and confidence as well as participants' self-reported integration of knowledge and skills into their practice. Implications for continuing education programs on suicide assessment and intervention are discussed.

For social workers, learning is not complete at the end of their formal social work education but needs to continue throughout their lifespan; via a process of lifelong learning, changes in knowledge, skills, and attitudes will likely occur (Lewis, 1998). Such learning can happen in many ways, including supervision, consultation, and continuing education participation (Simpson, Williams, & Segall, 2007). Continuing education programs create important structured opportunities for all practicing social workers to continue to learn new material related to a wide variety of social work topics, including new content areas and practice models (Congress, 2012; Nissen, Pendell, Jivanjee, & Goodluck, 2014). In recognition of the important role of continuing education, states require social workers to attend approved continuing education programs in order to maintain licensure. Yet, surprisingly, the social work education literature on the topic of effective continuing education is sparse (Nissen et al., 2014).

One content area in which many social workers identify a need for continuing education is suicide assessment and management (Feldman & Freedenthal,

2006; Singer & Slovak, 2011). In 2012, a National Strategy for Suicide Prevention report (U.S. Department of Health and Human Services, 2012) recognized a significant need to "provide training to mental health and substance abuse providers on the recognition, assessment and management of at-risk behavior, and the delivery of effective clinical care for people with suicide risk" (p. 46). In response to this call to action, several continuing education programs for mental health practitioners have been developed (Connor, Wood, Pisani, & Kemp, 2013; Cross, Gibbs, & White, 2011; Jacobson, Osteen, Jones, & Berman, 2012; Wharff, Ross, & Lambert, 2014). Given the importance of developing competence in assessing and managing suicide risk, evaluation of the effectiveness of these trainings in changing practitioners' knowledge, confidence, and behaviors is essential. This article describes the impact of one such training on participants' knowledge, confidence, and behaviors 3 months subsequent to the training.

Literature Review

In the United States, suicide is the 10th leading cause of death. In 2014, 42,773 people died by suicide (most recent data available; Centers for Disease Control, 2016). For every death by suicide, more than 20 emergency room visits are made due to suicidal ideation and behaviors and there are 25 suicide attempts (Centers for Disease Control, 2016). There is a significant need for mental health practitioners with the skills to effectively work with suicidal clients (Cramer, Johnson, McLaughlin, Rausch, & Conroy, 2013; Ruth, Gianino, Muroff, McLaughlin, & Feldman, 2012). Because social workers make up the largest group of professionals providing mental health services in the United States (Manderscheid & Berry, 2006; Weissman et al., 2006), suicide assessment and intervention is a relevant and important topic for social work education.

The experience of working with clients with suicidal ideation and behavior is a common one for many social workers. From an online survey of 598 social work practitioners, Feldman and Freedenthal (2006) found that 90% reported having worked with at least one client with suicidal ideation or behavior. Singer and Slovak (2011) found that this also was true for social workers placed in schools. In a survey of 399 school social workers, 88% reported working with a student with suicidal ideation or behavior and 64% with a student who had been hospitalized for this reason. Many social workers also experience a client's suicide attempt or death by suicide. A study of 515 social workers found that 55% reported working with at least one client who had made a suicide attempt (Sanders, Jacobson, & Ting, 2008). A national study of clinical social workers (N = 697) found that approximately one third had experienced a client's death by suicide (Jacobson, Ting, Sanders, & Harrington, 2004).

Social workers frequently work with clients with suicidal ideation and behavior (Jacobson et al., 2004; Sanders et al., 2008; Singer & Slovak, 2011), so it is somewhat surprising that social work graduate programs historically have given little space in the curriculum to suicide education (Feldman & Freedenthal, 2006; Ruth et al., 2012; Sanders et al., 2008). Although there are some exceptions, given that some social work schools have developed a graduate class on suicide or offer gatekeeper training on the assessment and management of at-risk clients (Jacobson et al., 2012; Scott, 2015), a survey of social work deans and directors found that few reported any intention of increasing suicide-related content in their curricula (Ruth et al., 2012). From a survey of advanced-year social work graduate students ($N = 73$), Osteen and colleagues (2014) found that students had just an average level of knowledge about working with clients with suicidal ideation and behavior and a low level of use of such knowledge with clients. Similarly, practicing social workers often report little confidence in their ability to work with suicidal clients (Feldman & Freedenthal, 2006; Singer & Slovak, 2011) and feel poorly prepared by their graduate programs for this type of clinical intervention (Sanders et al., 2008). Hence, there would appear to be a clear shortfall between the coverage of suicide education in social work graduate programs and the need in the field for knowledge, confidence, and skills in working with clients with suicidal ideation and behavior (Sanders et al., 2008). This gap makes continuing education on the topic an important issue for social work education; if social work students are not developing these skills in graduate school, then continuing education classes are needed for both recent graduates and more experienced practitioners in order for them to build necessary knowledge, confidence, and skills.

Multiple brief trainings on suicide assessment have been developed for social workers and other mental health professionals. The majority of them have been focused on teaching service providers to assess and support clients with suicidal thoughts and behaviors. Some of these programs have been geared toward social work students (Jacobson et al., 2012), whereas others primarily have been developed to fulfill a specific need, such as in the training of hospital social workers (Wharff et al., 2014). Several of these continuing education programs have demonstrated empirical support for their ability to improve knowledge and confidence around suicide assessment (Connor et al., 2013; Cross et al., 2011; Jacobson et al., 2012; Wharff et al., 2014). Coleman and Quest (2015) compared two of these trainings (Question, Persuade, Refer; RESPONSE) to a longer training (Applied Suicide Intervention Skills Trainings [ASIST]), which includes more emphasis on skill development. Although all three trainings demonstrated a change in attitudes toward suicide and feelings of self-efficacy, the participants of the longer training (ASIST) evidenced more significant changes in practice behaviors at the follow-up. Singer and Slovak (2011) suggested that practicing social workers (such as the school social workers in their sample) would most likely obtain the greatest benefit from a longer, skills-focused training such as ASIST. Several of these longer training programs, including ASIST (Rodgers, 2010), have demonstrated an ability to increase mental health professionals' knowledge and confidence in risk assessment and crisis intervention (Fenwick, Vassilas, Carter, & Haque, 2004; Gask, Dixon, Morriss, Appleby, & Green, 2006; Jacobson et al., 2012; Levitt, Lorenzo, Yu, Wean, & Miller-Solarino, 2011; Oordt, Jobes, Fonseca, & Schmidt, 2009). This outcome is especially likely when the training provides an opportunity for practicing skills, such as through role-plays (Cross et al., 2011). Nevertheless, more evaluation of clinical assessment and intervention trainings is needed to understand their effectiveness at teaching these complex skills to mental health practitioners and how service providers incorporate these skills into practice.

In recent years, the focus of social work education has evolved from knowledge learned to the development of practice competencies (Council on Social Work Education, 2015); the ability to apply knowledge and use skills is now a priority. This new emphasis reflects a growing recognition of the need for social workers not just to know information but to be able to translate that information into their practice with clients (Hackett, 2001; Nissen et al., 2014). When these ideas are applied to continuing education programs, program evaluation after the training needs to consider not just gains in knowledge and confidence but also a change in practice behavior, demonstrating that practitioners are successfully incorporating the new material into their practice. Rooney (1988) described three levels of effective learning for continuing education programs as (a) the acquisition of theory and skills, (b) the ability to demonstrate these skills by the end of the training, and (c) the ability to demonstrate these skills in practice. The majority of the evaluation in continuing education programs, however, is of Level 1 learning (Congress, 2012), which does not reflect the current emphasis in social work education on competencies. In the field of suicide prevention, this reality means that, although learning new material is important, changing mental health professionals' practice behaviors also is necessary (Oordt et al., 2009; Pisani, Cross, & Gould, 2011). Therefore, continuing education programs on suicide need to demonstrate that they can change behavior as well as enhance knowledge, attitudes, and confidence.

Evaluating behavior change can be complex and challenging. Nevertheless, several evaluations of continuing education programs have included behavioral change in their target outcomes. Oordt and colleagues (2009) followed up with clinicians ($N = 82$) 6 months after they attended the 12 hour Air Force Suicide Prevention Program and found that 83% of participants reported changing their suicide care practices with clients. Jacobson and colleagues (2012) used a case vignette to assess skill acquisition 4 months after the Recognizing and Responding to Suicide Risk training. Participants demonstrated increased skills in their responses to the vignette.

The aim of this research study was to determine the effectiveness of a newly developed 1-day continuing education program at maintaining increases of knowledge and confidence about suicide assessment and intervention, and changing participants' self-reported practice behaviors 3 months after the training.

Methods

Participants

A total of 598 participants attended a 6 hour continuing education workshop for mental health professionals titled Suicide Assessment and Intervention Training for Mental Health Professionals. Fourteen trainings were conducted at community agencies in Massachusetts from February 2013 to December 2014. There were 588 completed pretests, 514 completed posttests, and 237 completed 3-month follow-up questionnaires. (Of the follow-up questionnaires, 224 could be matched with pretests.)

Procedures

This study focuses on a 3-month follow-up of a one group pretest/posttest evaluation of the Suicide Assessment and Intervention Training for Mental Health Professionals workshop (formally known as Best Practices in Suicide Assessment and Intervention; Mirick, McCauley, Bridger & Berkowitz, 2016). As noted, the training is a 6 hour, 12-module continuing education workshop that addresses the core competencies in suicide risk assessment and management (Suicide Prevention Resource Center, 2006). See Table 1. Instructors use PowerPoint-guided lectures, practice exercises, role-plays, videos, writing activities, and discussions. This training covers assessment, crisis intervention, and a brief overview of treatment. Assessment includes

Table 1. Modules of the comprehensive approach to suicide assessment and crisis intervention training.

Module	Topic
Module #1	Understanding suicide
Module #2	Risk factors, warning signs & protective factors
Modules #3	Managing reactions
Module #4	Therapeutic empathy for the suicidal wish
Module #5	Eliciting the suicidal narrative
Module #6	Measures and tools for assessing level of risk
Module #7	Formulation of risk
Module #8	Crisis intervention and safety planning
Module #9	Best practices in treatment (Overview)
Module #10	Standard of care (liability, informed consent)
Module #11	Suicide postvention & working with survivors of suicide loss
Module #12	Self-care & Stories of hope

statistics about suicide, risk and protective factors, managing reactions, therapeutic empathy, eliciting the suicidal narrative, measures, and tools (including the Columbia Suicide Severity Rating Scale). Within the section on asking about suicidality, asking directly (e.g., asking, "Are you thinking about killing yourself?" vs. "Are you thinking about hurting yourself?") and validity techniques (e.g., gentle assumption, normalization, symptom amplification, shame attenuation, and behavioral incident) are discussed (Shea, 2002). Crisis interventions include means restriction, safety planning, using internal coping strategies (e.g., take a walk, listen to music), and external coping strategies (e.g., access friends, call counselor). Participants practice the development of a safety plan. The overview of treatment includes cognitive behavioral therapy, dialectical behavioral therapy, motivational interviewing, pharmacotherapy, and the use of online resources and applications. The training includes current evidence based practices, research, and statistics.

Initially, a one-group pretest/posttest research design was used to measure the impact of the training on participant knowledge and confidence. Participants completed anonymous pencil-and-paper pretests immediately before the training and posttests at the end of the training. This follow-up study, however, explores the retention of knowledge and confidence as well as self-reported behavior change. An anonymous Survey Monkey questionnaire was e-mailed to all participants ($N = 598$) 3 months subsequent to the training. The opportunity to enter a drawing for a $50 gift card was offered as an incentive to participate. Although the surveys were all anonymous, each participant was assigned a unique identification number so that pretests, posttests, and follow-up surveys could be matched.

Measures

Demographics and Work Experience
Demographic questions on the pretest asked about gender, work setting, profession, length of time in the field, number of clients with suicidal ideation or behaviors in the past 3 months, and number of previous suicide-related trainings.

Knowledge and Confidence
A questionnaire was used to measure knowledge and confidence. It consists of 25 questions using a 7-point Likert scale ranging from 7 (*strongly agree*) to 1 (*strongly disagree*). The instrument has strong face validity, and the internal consistency of this measure is good ($\alpha = 0.784$). This questionnaire was administered immediately before and immediately after the continuing education program as well as at the 3-month follow-up.

Behavior Change

Two open-ended questions asked, "Do you feel that you are using the knowledge and skills you learned in the training in your practice? and, If not, why not? If you answered yes, can you give an example of how you have used the knowledge or skills from the training in your practice?"

Data Management and Analyses

The data were entered into IBM SPSS Statistics for Windows, Version 21.0 (IBM, 2012), which was used to run all analyses. Posttests and follow-ups were matched with the original pretests whenever possible; in several instances the original, anonymous identification number was not included on the form, preventing a match from occurring. The responses were summed and scores were calculated for knowledge and confidence at pretest, posttest, and 3-month follow-up. Changes in knowledge and confidence from pretest to posttest, posttest to follow-up, and pretest to follow-up were assessed using three paired-sample t tests. Spearman rho correlations were run to look for relationships between participant variables (years of experience, number of trainings attended and number of clients in the past 3 months with suicidal ideation and/or behaviors) and pretest and follow-up knowledge and confidence. The primary researcher coded the open-ended responses. Only one rater was used, because little interpretation of the findings was required. For the first question, the majority of the responses were either yes or no. The coding for the second question was content coding; in their brief responses, most participants named the specific skills.

Results

Demographics

Demographics From Pretests Matched With Follow-Up

Although 237 follow-up questionnaires were completed, only 224 could be matched with completed pretests. Therefore, demographic data are available for only these 224 participants. The matched pretest/follow-up sample (n = 224) consisted of 171 (76.3%) women and 36 (16.1%) men (missing = 7.6%). There were 88 (39.3%) social workers, 60 (26.8%) mental health counselors, 41 (18.3%) psychologists, 12 (5.4%) nurses, and 22 (9.8%) who worked in other roles including art therapist, residential counselor, and marriage and family therapist (missing = 0.4%). Participants had an average of 11.65 years of experience in the field. They worked in a variety of settings: 73 (32.6%) in outpatient mental health centers, 53 (23.7%) in community agencies, 29 (12.9%) in schools, 15 (6.7%) in psychiatric emergency services, 10 (4.5%) in inpatient psychiatric settings, five (2.2%) in hospitals, nine

(4.0%) in residential programs, and the remaining 29 (13.0%) in a diversity of settings including the Department of Youth Services, day treatment programs, and private practice (missing = 0.4%). They had attended a mean of 1.92 previous suicide trainings and had worked with an average of 7.33 clients with suicidal ideation or behavior in the past 3 months (see Table 2).

Demographics of Pretests Not Matched With Follow-Up

The following demographic information is from the participants who completed pretests ($n = 588$), which could *not* be matched with a follow-up questionnaire ($n = 364$): There were 282 (77.5%) women and 63 (17.3%) men

Table 2. Comparison of Matched Pretest/Follow-Up Group to Unmatched Pretest Group

	Pretests not matched with follow-up[a]		Pretests matched with follow-up[b]			
	n (%)	M (SD)	n (%)	M (SD)	t (df/χ^2)	p
Pretest score	364	118.64 (16.09)	224	119.92 (16.29)	0.923 (467.54)	.356
Gender					0.066	.797
Male	63 (17.3)		36 (16.1)			
Female	282 (77.5)		171 (76.3)			
Missing	19 (5.2)		18 (8.0)			
Years of experience	356	12.07 (10.88)	219	11.65 (11.23)	0.443 (573)	.658
< 5 years	117 (32.1)		83 (37.1)			
≥ 5 years	239 (65.7)		136 (60.7)			
Missing	8 (2.2)		5 (2.2)			
Clients with suicidal ideation/ behavior (past 3 months)	355	8.94 (30.79)	224	7.33 (12.87)	0.740 (577)	.460
No clients	57 (15.7)		23 (10.3)			
≥ 1 client	298 (81.9)		201 (89.7)			
Missing	9 (2.5)		0 (0)			
No. of previous trainings	348	1.43 (2.10)	211	1.92 (4.18)	1.58 (278.18)	.114
No trainings	146 (40.7)		81 (33.8)			
≥ One training	202 (56.0)		130 (54.9)			
Not sure	10 (2.8)		8 (3.4)			
Missing	5 (1.4)		5 (2.2)			
Setting					16.281	.023
Outpatient	73 (20.1)		73 (32.6)			
Community agency	100 (27.5)		53 (23.7)			
School	71 (19.5)		29 (12.9)			
Emergency services	22 (6.0)		15 (6.7)			
Psychiatric inpatient	21 (5.8)		10 (4.5)			
Hospital	18 (5.0)		5 (2.2)			
Residential	16 (4.4)		9 (4.0)			
Other	43 (11.8)		29 (13.0)			
Missing	0 (0)		1 (0.5)			
Discipline					5.885	.208
Social work	135 (37.1)		88 (39.3)			
Counseling	92 (25.3)		60 (26.8)			
Psychology	56 (15.4)		41 (18.3)			
Nursing	35 (9.6)		12 (5.4)			
Other	46 (12.6)		22 (9.8)			
Missing	0 (0)		1 (0.5)			

[a]$n = 364$. [b]$n = 224$.

(missing = 19 [5.2%]), including 135 (37.1%) social workers, 92 (25.3%) mental health counselors, 56 (15.4%) psychologists, and 35 (9.6%) nurses. Participants had an average of 12.07 years of experience and worked in a variety of settings, including 73 (20.1%) in outpatient mental health centers, 100 (27.5%) in community agencies, 71 (19.5%) in schools, 22 (6.0%) in psychiatric emergency services, 21 (5.8%) in psychiatric inpatient, 18 (5.0%) in hospitals, 16 (4.4%) in residential programs, and the remaining 43 (11.8%) in other settings. They had attended a mean of 1.43 previous suicide trainings and had worked with an average of 8.94 clients with suicidal ideation and behavior in the past 3 months (see Table 2).

Comparison of Matched and Unmatched Pretest Demographics

As noted in Table 2, there was no significant difference in mean pretest score for the pretests that could be matched to posttests (M = 119.92, SD = 16.29) and those that could not (M = 118.64, SD = 16.09), t (471.28) = 0.923, p = .356, in years of experience for the matched pretests (M = 11.65, SD = 11.23) and those that were not (M = 12.07, SD = 10.88), $t(573)$ = 0.443, p = .658, in the number of clients in the past 3 months with suicidal ideation or behaviors for the matched pretests (M = 7.33, SD = 12.87) and those which were not (M = 8.94, SD = 30.79), $t(577)$ = 0.740, p = .460, or in the number of previous suicide trainings for matched pretests (M = 1.92, SD = 4.18) and those that were not (M = 1.43, SD = 2.10), $t(278.18)$ = 1.58, p = .114. There were no significant differences in discipline between the two groups (χ^2 = 5.885, p = .208). However, there was a significant association between the group and work setting (χ^2 = 16.281, p = .023).

Knowledge and Confidence

Among the 495 matched pretests and posttests, there was a significant increase in knowledge and confidence from pretest (M = 118.51, SD = 15.97) to posttest (M = 147.60, SD = 11.85), $t(494)$ = 44.98, p < .001. The effect size was moderate (0.719, Cohen's d = 2.069). There was a significant, positive relationship between pretest knowledge and confidence score and number of trainings (ρ = 0.475, p < .000, n = 557), number of clients with suicidal ideation and behaviors in the past 3 months (ρ = 0.230, p < .000, n = 568), and number of years of experience (ρ = 0.262, p < .000, n = 568).

A total of 237 three-month follow-up questionnaires were returned (a response rate of 40%), which included 224 matched pretests and follow-ups. There was a significant increase in the knowledge and confidence score from pretest (M = 119.92, SD = 16.29) to follow-up (M = 143.44, SD = 14.33, n = 224), $t(223)$ = 23.18, p < .001, with a moderate effect size (0.608, Cohen's

$d = 1.533$). The knowledge and confidence scores did decrease significantly from posttest ($M = 149.12$, $SD = 12.14$, $n = 215$) to follow-up ($M = 143.18$, $SD = 14.90$), $t(214) = 6.68$, $p < .001$, but the effect size was small (0.214, Cohen's $d = 0.437$). There was a weak, positive, significant relationship between follow-up knowledge and confidence scores and number of trainings previously attended ($\rho = 0.196$, $p = .004$, $n = 213$) and with the number of clients with suicidal ideation and behaviors seen in the past 3 months ($\rho = 0.159$, $p = .017$, $n = 223$) but no significant relationship with years of experience ($\rho = 0.116$, $p = .088$, $n = 218$). Further, a moderate, positive, significant relationship between the knowledge and confidence at the pretest and at the 3-month follow-up ($\rho = 0.539$, $p < .000$, $n = 224$) was found.

Use of Skills and Knowledge

Of the 237 participants who completed the 3-month follow-up questionnaire, 199 (84%) responded to the open-ended question "Do you feel that you are using the knowledge and skills you learned in the training in your practice?" One hundred seventy (85%) of those who responded said "yes," 22 (11%) responded "no," and seven (4%) responses were unclear or off-topic (see Table 3). Of those who responded "no," 11 (52%) said they were not currently practicing and seven (33%) said that they had not worked with any clients with suicidal ideation or behavior since the training. Ninety percent (153) of the participants who answered "yes" gave an example of how they had used the material from the training in their practice. Ninety-two (60%) participants said they used new skills in assessing clients; eleven (7%) of these participants specifically referenced the assessment tool introduced and practiced in the training (i.e., Columbia Suicide Severity Rating Scale). Forty-eight (31%) participants said they used the material by asking more direct, more frequent, and more detailed questions about suicidal ideation and behaviors (e.g., "Are you thinking about killing yourself?" instead of "Are you thinking of hurting yourself?"), and 23 (15%) reported

Table 3. Self-Report of Skills Used at 3-Month Follow-Up

Skills	n	%
Risk assessment	92	60
Use of assessment tools provided in training	11	7
Ask more frequent, more direct questions	48	31
Safety planning	23	15
Using safety planning in place of contracting for safety	5	3
Supporting staff at agency	7	5
Validity techniques	6	4
Changing agency protocols or programs	6	4
Other (e.g., supporting families, documentation, teaching coping skills, managing own reactions)	17	11

Note. $N = 153$. Total of percentages > 100 and n > 153 because participants gave more than one response.

using the newly learned material when conducting safety planning with clients.

Limitations

There are some limitations to the research design of this study. The presence of a pretest can affect the score on the posttest, or initial self-ratings of knowledge and confidence can be artificially high at pretest, before a thorough understanding of the topic has been developed. Without a control group, the exact impact of the pretest cannot be determined. To address this issue, future research might consider the use of a retrospective posttest paradigm (Pratt, 2000). With this design, no pretest is used; instead, at the end of the training, participants rate both their current knowledge and confidence, and their knowledge and confidence before the training. This design addresses both pretest sensitivity and response shift bias. Response bias represents another possible limitation, as there was an association between professional work setting and completed follow-up. Although there is no clear connection between setting and skill retention, it is possible that these differences affected the findings. In addition, a response rate of 40% raises the possibility that there may have been some subtle differences between the groups that impacted the process of learning or using knowledge and skills. There also were some challenges introduced by the use of anonymous identification numbers to match questionnaires over time; the ability to match all follow-ups to the correct pretests was lost due to the absence of an identification number or the use of an incorrect number. This made the comparison between the follow-up and non-follow-up groups more complicated. The evaluation of the acquisition of clinical skills is a challenging, complicated task, especially in community research. Clearly there are limitations to the use of self-report to measure outcomes. Although the anonymity of the surveys was designed to increase the likelihood of honest answers, it is possible that participants still gave artificially high scores or that their self-assessment, which involves perception, was inaccurate in some way. Moreover, this design does not control for any external events that may have occurred during the 3-month period; therefore, it is possible that some participants gained knowledge and confidence from some other source, such as an additional training. The addition of a control group in future research would address many of these limitations.

Discussion

Continuing education can be an effective approach for increasing social workers' knowledge and confidence around working with clients with suicidal ideation and behavior. In the current study, increased levels of knowledge and confidence were maintained for at least 3 months. Although knowledge and confidence scores went down slightly from the posttest scores, the effect size was low, and the follow-up scores remained significantly higher than the pretest scores. Participants who had attended a previous training on suicide had significantly higher pretest scores, suggesting that the impact of continuing education may last longer than just a few months. At the 3-month follow-up, although there was a positive relationship between previous number of trainings attended and score, the effect size was small ($\rho = 0.196$), much smaller than the correlation between number of trainings attended and the score at pretest ($\rho = 0.475$). It may be that although there is a small cumulative effect to attending multiple trainings on suicide (and it is certainly necessary from the perspective of remaining current on the research), a 1-day training is sufficient to impact knowledge and confidence substantially, even over time. Longer follow-up times would be needed to see if the impact of training on knowledge and confidence persists; in this study, participants were not asked the length of time since their last training. These findings support previous research which demonstrated that suicide assessment and intervention trainings can have an impact on knowledge and confidence that lasts for months, if not longer (Connor et al., 2013; Cross et al., 2011; Fenwick et al., 2004; Jacobson et al., 2012; Levitt et al., 2011; Oordt et al., 2009).

Nonetheless, recent work with clients experiencing suicidal ideation and behavior does not appear to have a strong relationship with follow-up levels of knowledge and confidence ($\rho = 0.159$). This finding is somewhat surprising, as the literature has shown that training participants learn knowledge and skills better if they have opportunities to practice the skills in the training, such as through role-play (Cross et al., 2011). Because opportunities to practice and use skills help develop and strengthen skill use, it would be logical to assume that mental health practitioners who do not have opportunities to use skills learned with clients will not retain the information as well. One possible explanation is that an assumption was made that the number of suicidal clients would remain fairly consistent over time. It may well be that, for many participants, the number of at-risk clients in their caseload varied substantially over time and that some of those with experience before the training did not have opportunities to use their new skills after the training, or vice versa. Participants' open-ended responses, however, suggest an alternative explanation. Several gave examples of using knowledge and skills that do not involve direct practice with clients with suicidal ideation or behavior, such as supporting staff at their agency through supervision (5%) and changing agency policies and protocols (4%). These participants described using the information and skills for "training my colleagues," "updating protocols," "creating safety plans," "supporting staff . . . in the wake of a suicide," and "developing a risk assessment protocol for my school." One participant, a faculty member, described how she incorporated material from the training, including a book and guest speaker, into her class to enhance her students' learning. Clearly, there are ways to share and use these skills with other professionals that do not involve direct work with clients and could create modest systemic change. Rudd, Cukrowicz, and Bryan (2008) highlighted the importance of the supervisory relationship for teaching suicide prevention skills, and Reeves, Wheeler, and Bowl (2004) found that individual supervision was an essential component of interns learning to assess and manage clients' suicidal thoughts and behaviors. In addition, a few participants reported using the material in outside-of-work venues, such as church and personal life. There may be multiple facets of participants' lives in which they can apply the material, which are unrelated to direct work with at-risk clients. This observation suggests that continuing education programs need not be aimed just at mental health practitioners working in direct practice. Explicitly talking about alternative ways to use these skills might help participants (such as teachers, trainers, and administrators) who are not directly working with clients conceptualize ways they could use the material in their other roles.

Not only did the continuing education program increase knowledge and confidence, more important, the majority of participants (85%) reported incorporating some of the knowledge and skills into their practice. This finding supports the ability of continuing education to fill in the gap between what is covered in social work programs and what is needed in the field (Feldman & Freedenthal, 2006; Osteen et al., 2014; Ruth et al., 2012; Singer & Slovak, 2011). Participants were most likely to report using assessment (60%) and assessment skills such as asking directly about suicide (31%) and validity techniques (4%). The only crisis intervention skill mentioned was safety planning, and that was by just 15% of respondents. This is somewhat surprising, as participants had an opportunity to practice safety planning in the training, which should increase retention of the skill (Cross et al., 2011).

Because Sanders et al. (2008) found that practicing social workers reported a need for more training specifically on "what to do" with clients experiencing suicidal thoughts and behaviors, the low numbers of participants who identified using safety-planning skills were unexpected. Some participants may not have needed to use crisis intervention skills if, after assessment, clients presented as low risk. Because assessment skills tend to be used more frequently than crisis intervention skills, the former may come to mind more quickly to participants than the latter. Baseline knowledge on current crisis interventions may be lower than for assessment. At the follow-up, five participants explicitly reported replacing their former practice of contracting for safety, an outdated intervention (Edwards & Sachmann, 2010), with safety planning.

Assessment skills also may be easier to learn and apply than crisis intervention skills. Assessment skills are a simpler set of skills that are often used to refer clients to higher intensity services (e.g., inpatient hospitalization, day treatment). Mental health practitioners often are overreliant on psychophar-macology and hospitalization (Jobes, Rudd, Overholser, & Joiner, 2008) and refer at-risk clients for evaluation instead of incorporating crisis intervention skills into their work. Although some at-risk clients require an inpatient level of care to maintain their safety, many do not and benefit more from ongoing crisis intervention work with their mental health practitioner.

Using crisis intervention skills can be more complex and requires the integration of knowledge as well as the management of the practitioner's own feelings. When working with at-risk clients, anxiety and fear often are high (Miller, McGlothlin, & West, 2013; Ting, Sanders, Jacobson, & Power, 2006). A 1-day training may not provide sufficient education and support for mental health practitioners to gain the required knowledge, confidence, and skills and to be able to manage their reactions to the work.

Future Research

In a review of suicide-related continuing education programs, Pisani et al. (2011) suggested that future research needs to explore how clinicians integrate material from continuing education programs into their practice. Although the findings of this study suggest that training participants are using the material from this particular training, they also highlight the continuing gap in the knowledge base. Indeed, at this point, little is known about how mental health professionals learn and apply material, especially intervention skills, taught in continuing education (Osteen et al., 2014; Webster-Wright, 2009). Further, this research study does not demonstrate which components of the training were particularly useful in encouraging mental health practitioners' changing practice behaviors. Although some aspects of the training likely played an important role—such as the emphasis on current evidence-based practices and managing reactions, as well as role-plays of assessment and safety planning—participants were not asked about the *process* of learning, which is a limitation of these findings.

To fill in this gap, research needs to explore social workers' perspectives on the content of continuing education programs and the process of applying the information learned (Ruth et al., 2012). Currently, the research that measures behavioral change tends to focus on the behavior but ignores the perspective and experience of the learner. Qualitative interviews with training participants could explore the process of integrat-ing knowledge and skills learned in the training into practice. Longitudinal follow-up research looking at outcomes of continuing education programs are needed as well to better understand the long-term impact of these trainings.

Conclusion

This study demonstrates the ability of a 1-day continuing education program to increase practitioners' knowledge and confidence when working with at-risk suicidal clients. In a context where social work graduate students may not be able to obtain sufficient training in the assessment and management of such at-risk clients (Feldman & Freedenthal, 2006; Ruth et al., 2012; Sanders et al., 2008), continuing education programs provide an important opportunity for practitioners to grow their knowledge and confidence. Schools of social work can take a leadership role in supporting the development and sustainability of such continuing education programs, as well as encouraging students, graduates, and faculty to access them in order to increase their knowledge, confidence, and skills in working with clients with suicidal ideation and behavior.

References

Centers for Disease Control and Prevention. (2016). *Leading causes of death, United States, 2013*. Retrieved from http://www.cdc.gov/nchs/fastats/suicide.htm

Coleman, D., & Quest, A. D. (2015). Science from evaluation: Testing hypotheses about differential effects of three youth-focused suicide prevention trainings. *Social Work in Public Health, 30*(2), 117–128. doi:10.1080/19371918.2014.938397

Congress, E. P. (2012). Guest editorial continuing education: Lifelong learning for social work practitioners and educators. *Journal of Social Work Education, 48*(3), 397–401. doi:10.5175/JSWE.2012.201200085

Connor, K. R., Wood, J., Pisani, A. R., & Kemp, J. (2013). Evaluation of a suicide prevention training curriculum for substance abuse treatment providers based on Treatment Improvement Protocol Number 50. *Journal of Substance Abuse Treatment, 44*, 13–16. doi:10.1016/j.jsat.201201.008

Council on Social Work Education. (2015). *Educational policy and accreditation standards*. Alexandria, VA: Author. Retrieved from http://www.cswe.org/File.aspx?id=81660

Cramer, R. J., Johnson, S. M., McLaughlin, J., Rausch, E. M., & Conroy, M. A. (2013). Suicide risk assessment training for psychology doctoral programs: Core competencies and a framework for training. *Training and Education in Professional Psychology, 7*(1), 1–11. doi:10.1037/a0031836

Cross, W. F., Gibbs, D., & White, A. (2011). Does practice make perfect? A randomized control trial of behavioral rehearsal on suicide prevention gatekeeper skills. *Journal of Primary Prevention, 32*, 195–211. doi:10.1007/s10935-011-0250-z

Edwards, S. J., & Sachmann, M. D. (2010). No-suicide contracts, no-suicide agreements, and no-suicide assurances: A study of their nature, utilization, perceived effectiveness and potential to cause harm. *Crisis: The Journal of Crisis Intervention and Suicide Prevention, 31*(6), 290–302. doi:10.1027/0227-5910/a000048

Feldman, B. N., & Freedenthal, S. (2006). Social work education in suicide intervention and prevention: An unmet need? *Suicide and Life Threatening Behavior, 36*, 467–480. doi:10.1521/suli.2006.36.issue-4

Fenwick, C. D., Vassilas, C. A., Carter, H., & Haque, M. S. (2004). Training health professionals in the recognition, assessment and management of suicide risk.

International Journal of Psychiatry in Clinical Practice, 8, 117–121. doi:10.1080/13651500410005658

Gask, L., Dixon, C., Morriss, R., Appleby, L., & Green, G. (2006). Evaluating STORM skills training for managing people at risk of suicide. *Journal of Advanced Nursing, 54,* 739–750. doi:10.1111/jan.2006.54.issue-6

Hackett, S. (2001). Educating for competency and reflective practice: Fostering a conjoint approach in education and training. *Journal of Workplace Learning, 13,* 103–112. doi:10.1108/13665620110388406

IBM Corporation. (2012). *IBM SPSS Statistics for Windows, Version 21.0.* Armonk, NY: IBM Corporation.

Jacobson, J. M., Osteen, P., Jones, A., & Berman, A. (2012). Evaluation of the recognizing and responding to suicide risk training. *Suicide and Life-Threatening Behavior, 42*(5), 471–485. doi:10.1111/j.1943-278X.2012.00105.x

Jacobson, J. M., Ting, L., Sanders, S., & Harrington, D. (2004). Prevalence of and reactions to fatal and nonfatal clients' suicidal behavior: A national study of mental health social workers. *Omega: Journal of Death and Dying, 49,* 237–248.

Jobes, D. A., Rudd, M. D., Overholser, J. C., & Joiner, T. E. (2008). Ethical and competence care of suicidal patients: Contemporary challenges, new developments and considerations for clinical practice. *Professional Psychology: Research and Practice, 39*(4), 405–413. doi:10.1037/a0012896

Levitt, A. J., Lorenzo, J., Yu, V., Wean, C., & Miller-Solarino, S. (2011). Teaching Note: Suicide awareness and prevention workshop for social workers and paraprofessionals. *Journal of Social Work Education, 47*(3), 607–615. doi:10.5175/JSWE.2011.200900108

Lewis, M. (1998). Lifelong learning: Why professionals must have the desire for and the capacity to continue learning throughout life. *Health Information Management, 28,* 62–66.

Manderscheid, R. W., & Berry, J. T. (2006). *Mental health, United States, 2004* (DHHS Publ. No. 06-4195). Rockville, MD: Substance Abuse and Mental Health Services Administration, Center for Mental Health Services. Retrieved from http://store samhsa. gov/shin/content/SMA06-4195/SMA06-4195.pdf

Miller, L. G., McGlothlin, J. M., & West, J. D. (2013). Taking the fear out of suicide assessment and intervention: A pedagogical and humanistic practice. *The Journal of Humanistic Counseling, 52*(1), 106–121. doi:10.1002/johc.2013.52.issue-1

Mirick, R. G., McCauley, J., Bridger, J., & Berkowitz, L. (2016). Continuing education on suicide assessment and crisis intervention: What can we learn about the needs of mental health professionals in community practice? *Community Mental Health Journal, 52,* 501–510.

Nissen, L., Pendell, K., Jivanjee, P., & Goodluck, C. (2014). Lifelong learning in social work education: A review of the literature and implications for the future. *Journal of Teaching in Social Work, 34,* 384–400. doi:10.1080/08841233.2014.936577

Oordt, M. S., Jobes, D. A., Fonseca, V. P., & Schmidt, S. M. (2009). Training mental health professionals to assess and manage suicidal behavior: Can provider confidence and practice behaviors be altered? *Suicide and Life-Threatening Behavior, 39,* 21–32. doi:10.1521/suli.2009.39.1.21

Osteen, P. J., Jacobson, J. M., & Sharpe, T. L. (2014). Suicide prevention in social work education: How prepared are social work students? *Journal of Social Work Education, 50,* 349–364.

Pisani, A. R., Cross, W. F., & Gould, M. S. (2011). The assessment and management of suicide risk: State of workshop education. *Suicide and Life-Threatening Behavior, 41*(3), 255–276. doi:10.1111/j.1943-278X.2011.00026.x

Pratt, C.C. (2000). Measuring program outcomes: Using retrospective pretest methodology. *American Journal of Evaluation, 21*, 341–349.

Reeves, A., Wheeler, S., & Bowl, R. (2004). Assessing risk: Confrontation or avoidance—What is taught on counselor training courses? *British Journal of Guidance and Counseling, 32*, 235–247. doi:10.1080/03069880410001697288

Rodgers, P. (2010). *Review of the Applied Suicide Intervention Skills training Program (ASIST): Rationale, evaluation results, and directions for future research.* Retrieved from http://iers.umt.edu/docs/msscdocs/ASIST_review2010.pdf

Rooney, R. H. (1988). Measuring task-centered training effects on practice: Results of an audiotape study in a public agency. *Journal of Continuing Social Work Education, 4*(4), 2–7.

Rudd, M. D., Cukrowicz, K. C., & Bryan, C. J. (2008). Core competencies in suicide risk assessment and management: Implications for supervision. *Training and Education in Professional Psychology, 2*(4), 219–228. doi:10.1037/1931-3918.2.4.219

Ruth, B. J., Gianino, M., Muroff, J., McLaughlin, D., & Feldman, B. N. (2012). You can't recover from suicide: Perspectives on suicide education in MSW programs. *Journal of Social Work Education, 48*(3), 501–516. doi:10.5175/JSWE.2012.201000095

Sanders, S., Jacobson, J. M., & Ting, L. (2008). Preparing for the inevitable: Training social workers to cope with client suicide. *Journal of Teaching in Social Work, 28*(1/2), 1–18. doi:10.1080/08841230802178821

Scott, M. (2015). Teaching note—Understanding of suicide prevention, intervention, and postvention: Curriculum for MSW students. *Journal of Social Work Education, 51*, 177–185. doi:10.1080/10437797.2015.979095

Shea, S. (2002). *The practical art of suicide assessment: A guide for mental health professionals and substance abuse counselors.* New York, NY: Wiley & Sons.

Simpson, G. A., Williams, J. C., & Segall, A. B. (2007). Social work education and clinical learning. *Clinical Social Work Journal, 35*, 3–14. doi:10.1007/s10615-006-0046-4

Singer, J. B., & Slovak, K. (2011). School social workers' experiences with youth suicidal behavior: An exploratory study. *Children & Schools, 33*, 215–229. doi:10.1093/cs/33.4.215

Suicide Prevention Resource Center. (2006). *Core competencies in the assessment and management of suicidality.* Newton, MA: Author.

Ting, L., Sanders, S., Jacobson, J. M., & Power, J. R. (2006). Dealing with the aftermath: A qualitative analysis of mental health social workers' reactions after a client suicide. *Social Work, 51*(4), 329–341. doi:10.1093/sw/51.4.329

U.S. Department of Health and Human Services Office of the Surgeon General and National Action Alliance for Suicide Prevention. (2012). *National Strategy for Suicide Prevention: Goals and Objectives for Action.* Washington, DC: U.S. Department of Health and Human Services.

Webster-Wright, A. (2009). Reframing professional development through understanding authentic professional learning. *Review of Educational Research, 79*(2), 702–739. doi:10.3102/0034654308330970

Weissman, M. M., Verdeli, H., Gameroff, M. J., Bledsoe, S. E., Betts, K., Mufson, L., ... Wickramaratne, P. (2006). National survey of psychotherapy training in psychiatry, psychology and social work. *Archives of General Psychiatry, 63*, 925–934. doi:10.1001/archpsyc.63.8.925

Wharff, E. A., Ross, A. M., & Lambert, S. (2014). Field note—Developing suicide risk assessment training for hospital social workers: An academic-community partnership. *Journal of Social Work Education, 50*, 184–190. doi:10.1080/10437797.2014.856249

The Learning Institute: Promoting Social Justice Advocacy Within a Continuing Education Program

Karen Rice, Heather Girvin, Jennifer Frank, and Leonora Foels

ABSTRACT

The pursuit of social justice is an overarching framework that defines the social work profession. The goals of macro social work practice are centered on issues of social justice with strategies that include changing community conditions and creating a sense of solidarity, with particular emphasis on broadening the opportunities for marginalized populations. Given the natural alignment between social justice and macro social work practice, the exclusion of macro practice content in educational experiences should concern social workers and educators alike. The Learning Institute emerged in large part from a school's shared concern with the micro/macro dichotomy that often characterizes the profession, as well as the faculty's commitment to renewing the profession's dedication to our social justice mandate. Results from this formative assessment clearly suggest that participants in the Learning Institute series may have experienced bifurcated education, exposure, and training to social justice advocacy on the macrolevel. Implications for future research and continuing education are discussed.

The National Association of Social Workers (1999) has asserted that the pursuit of social justice is an overarching responsibility that defines our profession's work. The Council on Social Work Education (2015) supported this mandate, requiring that social work education provide ample opportunities for students to develop competence related to advocacy and the pursuit of social equity. Despite the professional and educational endorsement of the *idea* of social justice, and the explicit articulation of this objective as our profession's distinguishing characteristic, education and training related to social justice and social equity have been relegated to a secondary position in many social work program curricula, and professional trends suggest that real-world practice may have lost sight of this mandate, as well (Ferguson, 2008; Van Voorhis & Hostetter, 2006). However, students have not abandoned their interest in social justice and, in fact, see their professional function as vital to the confrontation of social injustices and oppression (Findlay & McCormack, 2007; Rotabi, Gammonley, Gamble, & Weil, 2007).

Indeed, it seems that their interest is keen and their awareness of their social justice obligation is infused with pride. The challenge, however, is that course content typically meets this interest at the "value level," underscoring the importance of social justice but failing to provide content that specifically addresses interventions for effective macro practice driven by principles of social justice (Aponte, 1995; Schmitz, Stakeman, & Sisneros, 2001).

Postsecondary professional development could offer opportunities to offset these trends. Continuing education (universally required now for social work licensure renewal) could address the dearth of training related to both macro-level practice and social justice. Nevertheless, typical continuing education offerings reflect current professional trends: They focus on direct-practice, microlevel intervention strategies and/or raise issues related to diversity but fall short of providing adequate macrolevel intervention strategies, instead emphasizing the development of effective micro practice skills in the context of an increasingly diverse client population (Schmitz et al., 2001).

Literature Review

Over the years, social work has struggled with establishing a consistent and coherent professional identity. In part, the difficulty can be traced to the divergent roots of the profession (Austin, Coombs, & Barr, 2005; Epple, 2007). Although the Charity Organization Society (COS) and the Settlement House Movement (SHM) both sought to deal with the issues of those experiencing societal oppression, they did so from very different viewpoints.

The casework performed by "friendly visitors" exemplified the application of Scientific Charity (Speizman, 1965). Through this modality, the COS attempted to provide a systematic method for professionally assessing the needs of the disadvantaged. Although labeling the COS as paternalistic often undermines the genuineness of their motivations, the work of the COS has been noted for its primary focus on the individual and as the precursor to micro clinical practice.

Conversely, the SHM emphasized the power of recognizing the collective good through its focus on community building and empowerment. In the context of functional communities, where diversity and strengths were celebrated, the SHM focused on creating broader societal changes in light of the needs of the groups with whom they worked (Netting, Kettner, & McMurtry, 2008). The work of the SHM has been touted for its primary focus on the community and as the precursor to community-based macro practice.

False Dichotomy

Although the COS is oft cited as the root of the micro arm of the social work profession, its attempts to systematize aid through a process of community collaboration cannot solely be construed as microlevel work. In addition to the use of individual casework, the COS sought to coordinate pockets of charitable aid within the community (Netting et al., 2008; Speizman, 1965). Although the desire to add consistency and rigor to methods of decision making in applying aid was to help ensure that the "imposter" would not usurp an unwarranted portion of already-limited community resources, these were markedly macro-type activities (Netting et al., 2008). Similarly, although the SHM is often heralded as the root of macro social work, work with individuals in the context of residential communities, using micro skills and case advocacy, was always present. Further, although the divide in the social work profession often has been traced to these divergent professional origins, the educational setting (Shdaimah & McCoyd, 2012) and contemporary practice narratives (Vodde & Galiant, 2002) may have further reified this divide.

Fostering the Divide

In addition to the common narrative just cited, regarding the origins of the profession, the great divide between micro and macro work is fostered through social work education and professional terminology. According to Austin et al. (2005), the tension and strain between micro and macro social work practice has been "perpetuated in agencies and academia" (p. 27). Indeed, social work educators often are situated in opposing camps and identified as micro, to the exclusion of macro, or vice versa (Shdaimah & McCoyd, 2012). Articulated divisions and obvious omissions in curricula clearly accentuate this divide (Specht & Courtney, 1994).

Common uses of professional terminology also have contributed to these professional divisions. According to Hill, Ferguson, and Erickson (2010), social workers engaging in macro activities tend not to embrace social work as a professional identity but rather opt for the titles specific to the work they do (e.g., community organizer, policy analyst). Similarly, social workers engaged in micro work frequently choose to identify themselves as clinicians or therapists. These titles tend to further divide the profession.

Why a Focus on Micro Causes Concern

Not only does the lack of integration and continuity between the micro and macro professional bookends raise cause for concern, but also there often is a real or perceived bias in favor of micro practice (and clinical modalities) to the exclusion of macro practice (Specht & Courtney, 1994). According to Hill et al. (2010), macro practice frequently is not viewed as the central focus of either social work practice or social work education. Calling this phenomenon an "imbalance," Rothman and Mizrahi (2014) observed that efforts are being made (and should be made) to promote the application of macro work in the classroom and in the field (p. 91).

In their discussion of an innovative model for teaching macro practice to social work students, Edmonds-Cady and Sosulski (2012) highlighted specific challenges to teaching and emphasizing macro work, such as the nonlinear fashion of social change, the difficult work of creating community relationships, and the time constraints embedded in the academic calendar. The result is a focus on micro work, where skills are easier to practice in the context of the classroom. Nevertheless, to prepare future social workers, proper training in macro practice today is essential (Edmonds-Cady & Sosulski, 2012). According to Specht and Courtney (1994), dealing with individuals through primarily individual psychotherapy fails to consider contextual factors that contribute to ongoing social injustice.

The social work profession's ethical commitment to social justice (National Association of Social Workers, 1999) requires social work educators and practitioners to keep a watchful eye on structures in society that may serve to marginalize the vulnerable (Bent-Goodley, 2014). Looking back, both the COS and SHM held high that same definition and vision of social justice. As social workers, we naturally must be concerned about any division or imbalance that compromises the integrity of our social justice mandate.

Integration of Micro and Macro for Social Justice

Given the natural alignment between social justice and macro social work practice, the exclusion of macro practice content in educational experiences should give pause and concern to social workers and educators alike. Austin and colleagues (2005) suggested that the person-in-environment perspective, which dates back to the work of the settlement house movement, is the common thread between the micro and macro foci of the profession. Vodde and Galiant (2002) cited Mills's (1959) call for a connection between the micro and macro (using the "sociological imagination") and suggested a model to blend the two. Rothman and Mizrahi (2014) have issued a call for action in balancing micro and macro practice, as well.

The Learning Institute: Global Well-Being and Social Change

In 2013, the Millersville University School of Social Work in Pennsylvania launched its continuing education program, titled The Learning Institute: Global Well-Being and Social Change, in an effort to promote global citizenship by raising awareness around social issues and enhancing advocacy skills in order to foster social justice. From survey data, each year a theme is chosen to guide the planning of the Learning Institute events. These themes reflect the Learning Institute's dedication to social justice and have included youth violence, sexual exploitation of women and children, and poverty and human need. In calls for proposals and related materials, these issues are framed as ones that are shared but differentially experienced by marginalized groups from around the world. The Learning Institute hosts monthly continuing education workshops and trainings that align with the theme and offers these to students, educators, and community members.

In addition to offering continuing education units that can be applied toward licensure renewal, the intent of the Learning Institute is to offer knowledge and skills that will support all levels of social work practice. Early in the year, the continuing education events tend to be knowledge based, and progress to skill development, with content that reflects micro, mezzo, and macro advocacy and interventions. The yearlong events culminate at the end of the academic year, followed by an international conference in early summer with local, state, national, and international participants. This conference is used to reinforce the Learning Institute's global framework and its commitment to global citizenship and social justice. In addition to a keynote and plenary speaker, there are a number of continuing education workshops from which participants may choose. Presentations reflect content related to the selected theme and depict the varying manifestations of the same social issue across the globe.

The Learning Institute emerged in large part from the school's shared concern with the micro/macro dichotomy that characterizes the profession, as well as the faculty's commitment to renewing the profession's dedication to social justice. This study summarizes data gathered to explore this concern. Next we discuss findings and their role in shaping the Learning Institute's future planning.

Method

Sample

The sample comprises 69 individuals who participated in the first Learning Institute's monthly events, excluding the annual conference, during the 2013–14 academic year and who chose to complete the survey following each event. Ninety-nine total individuals participated in the events, thus the sample size of 69 represents a 70% response rate. Participants (see Table 1) were predominantly students ($n = 6$, 81.2%), women ($n = 61$, 88.4%), non-Hispanic/Latino ($n = 58$, 84.1%), White/Caucasian ($n = 50$, 73.5%), and on average 25 years old ($SD = 9.01$). (The 13 nonstudents comprised educators and practitioners.) The students represent graduate and undergraduate students from across many disciplines, including but not limited to social work, psychology, sociology, criminology, and international studies.

Data Collection

Individuals who participated in the initial Learning Institute's events were provided a survey upon registering for the continuing education training

Table 1. Sample Demographics.

Demographics	N	%
Educational status		
Student	56	81.2%
Nonstudent	13	18.8%
Gender		
Male	8	11.6%
Female	61	88.4%
Ethnicity		
Hispanic/Latino	10	14.5%
Non-Hispanic/Non-Latino	58	84.1%
Race		
Black/African American	11	16.2%
White/Caucasian	50	73.5%
Native American	3	4.4%
Asian American	1	1.5%
Other	3	4.4%

Note. Difference in total sample size is due to participants choosing not to respond to questions related to ethnicity and race. Age $M = 25$ ($SD = 9.01$).

and asked to complete it and hand it in by the end of the 1-hour presentation. Completion of the survey was voluntary, and those who chose to participate deposited it in a box as they exited the venue. Approval to conduct the study was obtained from the university's Institutional Review Board, and confidentiality was maintained to avoid identifying the individual completing the survey. The instrument comprised 12 demographic questions (e.g., gender, race, age, education status) and the Social Justice Advocacy Scale (Dean, 2009). There are four subscales that compose the overall Social Justice Advocacy Scale: Collaborative Action ($\alpha = .92$), Social/Political Advocacy ($\alpha = .91$), Client Empowerment ($\alpha = .76$), and Client/Community Advocacy ($\alpha = .76$). The scale comprises 43 questions with Likert-style response options ranging from 1 (*not at all true*) to 7 (*totally true*). The Collaborative Action subscale comprises 20 questions and measures the degree to which participants build relationships with community groups and social justice advocates, as well as raise their awareness about social injustices. The Social/Political Advocacy subscale, comprising seven questions, measures the degree to which participants engage in social/political advocacy to influence political processes or public policy toward socially just legislation. Eight questions make up the Client Empowerment subscale, which measures the degree to which participants have the ability to identify the effects of social injustices on clients and their ability to help the client to develop skills for self-advocacy. The final subscale, Client/Community Advocacy, assesses the degree to which participants use their advocacy skills to benefit the client and the extent to which they understand how social issues affect their client. Eight questions make up this fourth subscale.

Table 2. Internal Reliability Consistency.

Social Justice Advocacy subscales	á
Collaborative Action	.922
Social/Political Advocacy	.817
Client Empowerment	.618
Client/Community Advocacy	.592

Data Analysis

Cronbach's alpha was performed to assess internal reliability consistency (see Table 2). Descriptive statistics were performed to conduct a formative assessment of individuals' commitments to macro practice and social justice advocacy, as operationalized by the Social Justice Advocacy Scale. Further, independent sample t tests were conducted to determine whether there were any mean differences in outcome variables (four subscales) between students and nonstudents.

Results

Two of the four subscales were found to be in the suitable range ($\alpha = .70$ or above) as recommended by de Vaus (2009). The other two, although less than .70, show acceptable internal reliability, ranging from .592 to .618.

Table 3 displays the findings of participants' overall mean on each subscale. The means range from a high of 5.79 ($SD = .85$) for Client/Community Advocacy to a low of 2.89 ($SD = 1.34$) for Social/Political Advocacy.

There was no statistically significant difference between students and nonstudents on either outcome variable (see Table 4): Collaborative Action ($t = -1.32$, $p = .193$), Social/Political Advocacy ($t = -1.51$, $p = .136$), Client Empowerment ($t = -.599$, $p = .551$), Client/Community Advocacy ($t = .719$, $p = .475$).

Table 3. Group Mean Outcomes.

Social Justice Advocacy subscales	M	SD
Collaborative Action	3.68	1.25
Social/Political Advocacy	2.89	1.34
Client Empowerment	4.71	1.98
Client/Community Advocacy	5.79	0.85

Table 4. Outcome Differences Between Students and Nonstudents.

Social Justice Advocacy subscales	Student			Nonstudent				
	N	M	SD	N	M	SD	t	p
Collaborative Action	49	3.58	1.17	11	4.13	1.54	−1.32	.193
Social/Political Advocacy	50	2.76	1.23	12	3.40	1.68	−1.51	.163
Client Empowerment	50	4.64	2.11	12	5.02	1.36	−.599	.551
Client/Community Advocacy	47	5.83	0.86	11	5.63	0.80	.719	.475

Discussion

The purpose of this study was to assess students' current focus on macro social work practice and the incorporation of our profession's social justice mandate into their work. Further, the study explored whether there was a difference between students and nonstudents with respect to these outcomes.

Results from this formative assessment suggest that participants in the Learning Institute series may have experienced the bifurcated education, exposure, and training as just described, as participants acknowledged engaging more in client empowerment and client/community advocacy (microlevel advocacy) rather than in collaborative action and social/political advocacy (macrolevel advocacy). Ferguson (2008) warned that in order for our profession to thrive, we must reclaim our social justice mandate and rediscover our humanity. Therefore, the need for increased training related to advocacy and social justice seems clear. As our postsecondary educational institutions struggle to accommodate an advocacy and social justice mandate, it may well be that continuing education programs offer promising avenues to address the micro/macro split and return advocacy and social justice to the center of social work practice.

It would be inaccurate, however, to suggest that social work curricula are bereft of social justice advocacy content. Kam Kwong (2012) reminded us that social justice and its links to practice remain present in BSW and MSW curricula; however, the link is predominately between social justice and micro practice. For many students, the clinical leanings of the curricula and their own lack of real-world experiences may coalesce to foster an overattentiveness to social justice concerns as reflected in direct micro practice. O'Brien (2010) echoed this characterization of social work education and stated that social workers' social justice advocacy has been weak in public policy and social change. Our own research findings reflect these trends.

Continuing education events hosted by the Learning Institute offset the perceived micro bias of the social work curricula. Invited speakers and scholarly presenters were vetted through a global social justice lens (e.g., presenters were asked to frame their workshops utilizing a social justice lens). Students bring their often newly acquired social justice frame of reference, and practitioners provide a lived perspective. As students and practitioners interact in the context of events, a mutually beneficial synergy occurs. Practitioners are reminded of the importance of social justice advocacy, and students are provided with real-life examples of structural barriers at macro/mezzo levels that require systemic advocacy. The potential of creating opportunities for collaborative learning between students and practitioners of course is not a new idea. Lundy (2004) argued that organizations (such as the Learning Institute) need to take leadership roles in aiding professionals by linking their daily activities to social justice advocacy. Optimally, at Learning Institute continuing education events, practitioners are reengaged by students who are passionately committed to social justice, and students learn to operationalize and implement their ideals through interactions with seasoned professional practitioners.

Further study is required to assess the extent to which we see increases in scores for participants in the Learning Institute events, especially along measures of collaborative action (building relationships with community groups for social justice advocacy) and social/political advocacy. Additional research also should explore the degree to which learning comes from the content of the Learning Institute Continuing Education events, and/or the interaction between the students and professionals, and whether lessons learned for these two cohorts differ.

Implications for Social Work Continuing Education

Results from this study would tend to support the need for more continuing education programs focusing on the integration of micro/macro social work practice, specifically the mandate to promote social justice advocacy. Such advocacy is relevant to a global society (Helms, 2003) because it is essential for us to engage in critical dialogue around both the prosperity and devastation caused by globalization. As Smith and Cheung (2015) remind us, this training is essential because social workers can utilize the knowledge and skills gleaned to promote more effective decision making and resource allocation.

The Learning Institute is oriented toward global issues, with the understanding that many social problems that affect "us" also affect "them." The Learning Institute model is to work to close the gap in dichotomous thinking. According to Corbett and Fikkert (2012), the Western tendency to create dichotomies has resulted in the marginalization of groups, as well as in the artificial bifurcation of our intervention strategies between micro/macro. It seems plausible that a refocusing on global social issues—and our shared involvement in them—may provide a conceptual framework for training related to advocacy and social justice across all levels of practice, and continuing education may be one remedy that will prove to be as comprehensive as the need.

References

Aponte, C. L. (1995). Cultural diversity course model: Cultural competence for content and process. *Arete, 20*, 46–55.

Austin, M., Coombs, M., & Barr, B. (2005). Community-centered clinical practice: Is the integration of micro and macro social work practice possible? *Journal of Community Practice, 13*(4), 9–30. doi:10.1300/J125v13n04_02

Bent-Goodley, T. (2014). Social work practice: Innovation and social justice for a changing world. *Social Work, 59*(2), 101–102. doi:10.1093/sw/swu006

Corbett, S., & Fikkert, B. (2012). *When helping hurts: How to alleviate poverty without hurting the poor . . . and yourself.* Chicago, IL: Moody.

Council on Social Work Education. (2015). *Educational policy and accreditation standards.* Alexandria, VA: Author.

Dean, J. K. (2009). *Quantifying social justice advocacy competency: Development of the social justice advocacy scale.* (Unpublished Doctoral Dissertation). Received from http://digitalarc hive.gsu.edu/cps_diss/40

de Vaus, D. (2009). *Analyzing social science data: 50 key problems in data analysis.* Thousand Oaks, CA: Sage.

Edmonds-Cady, C., & Sosulski, M. (2012). Applications of situated learning to foster communities of practice. *Journal of Social Work Education, 48*(1), 45–64. doi:10.5175/JSWE.2012.201000010

Epple, D. (2007). Inter and intra professional social work differences: Social work's challenge. *Clinical Social Work Journal, 35,* 267–276. doi:10.1007/s10615-007-0098-0

Ferguson, I. (2008). *Reclaiming social work: Challenging neo-liberalism and promoting social justice.* Thousand Oaks, CA: Sage.

Findlay, M., & McCormack, J. (2007). Globalization and social work education and practice: Exploring Australian practitioners' views. *Journal of Sociology and Social Welfare, 34,* 123–142.

Helms, J. E. (2003). A pragmatic view of social justice. *The Counseling Psychologist, 31,* 305–313. doi:10.1177/0011000003031003006

Hill, K., Ferguson, S., & Erickson, C. (2010). Sustaining and strengthening a macro identity: The association of macro practice social work. *Journal of Community Practice, 18,* 513–527. doi:10.1080/10705422.2010.519684

Kam Kwong, P. (2012). Back to the 'social' of social work: Reviving the social work profession's contribution to the promotion of social justice. *International Social Work, 57,* 723–740.

Lundy, C. (2004). *Social work and social justice.* Ontario, Canada: Broadview Press.

Mills (1959). *The sociological imagination.* New York, NY: Oxford University Press.

National Association of Social Workers. (1999). *Code of ethics.* Washington, DC: Author.

Netting, F., Kettner, P., & McMurtry, S. (2008). *Social work macro practice* (4th ed.). New York, NY: Pearson.

O'Brien, M. (2010). Social justice: Alive and well (partly) in social work practice? *International Social Work, 54,* 174–190. doi:10.1177/0020872810382682

Rotabi, K. S., Gammonley, D., Gamble, D. N., & Weil, M. O. (2007). Integrating globalization into the social work curriculum. *Journal of Sociology and Social Welfare, 34,* 165–185.

Rothman, J., & Mizrahi, T. (2014). Balancing micro and macro practice: A challenge for social work. *Social Work, 59*(1), 91–93. doi:10.1093/sw/swt067

Schmitz, C. L., Stakeman, C., & Sisneros, J. (2001). Educating professionals for practice in a multicultural society: Understanding oppression and valuing diversity. *Families in Society: The Journal of Contemporary Social Services, 82,* 612–622. doi:10.1606/1044-3894.160

Shdaimah, C., & McCoyd, J. (2012). Social work sense and sensibility: A framework for teaching an integrated perspective. *Social Work Education, 31*(1), 22–35. doi:10.1080/02615479.2010.541237

Smith, D. S., & Cheung, M. (2015). Research note—Globalization and social work: Influencing practice through continuing education. *Journal of Social Work Education, 51,* 583–594.

Specht, H., & Courtney, M. (1994). *Unfaithful angels: How social work has abandoned its mission.* New York, NY: The Free Press.

Speizman, M. (1965). Poverty, pauperism, and their cases: Some charity organization views. *Social Casework, 46,* 142–149.

Van Voorhis, R. M., & Hostetter, C. (2006). The impact of MSW education on social worker empowerment and commitment to client empowerment through social justice advocacy. *Journal of Social Work Education, 42,* 105–121. doi:10.5175/JSWE.2006.200303147

Vodde, R., & Galiant, J. (2002). Bridging the gap between micro and macro practice: Large scale change and a unified model of narrative-deconstructive practice. *Journal of Social Work Education, 38,* 439–458.

A Gerontology Practitioner Continuing Education Certificate Program: Lessons Learned

Jacqueline Englehardt, Kristina M. Hash, Mariann Mankowski, Karen V. Harper-Dorton, and Ann E. Pilarte

ABSTRACT

This article discusses the results of a school of social work survey assessing the geriatric training needs of social workers and other professionals in aging and the need for a gerontology practitioner's continuing education (CE) certificate program. A total of 391 professionals, the majority of whom were social workers, participated in an online needs assessment survey. Of all respondents, the majority (77%) expressed some interest in enrolling in a certificate program within 2 years. Increased knowledge and competence, personal satisfaction and growth, and meeting CE requirements for professional licensure renewal were the major reasons given for interest in enrollment. Cognitive changes, dementia, and end-of-life issues were each selected by almost half of the respondents as areas in which they felt they needed the most training. Legal issues, health care, and social policies and programs were also of interest. In response to survey findings, a 100-clock-hour program was developed to strengthen the skills of persons who work with older adults. The emphasized curricular areas included understanding aging processes and social and economic issues confronting older persons. Related programs, seeking to assess the geriatric training needs of professionals in efforts to develop an appropriate educational program to respond to these needs, can benefit from challenges and lessons learned from this interdisciplinary CE program development.

Introduction

The United States is experiencing an unprecedented number of persons reaching and surpassing the age of 65; in fact, the population of those 65 and older is expected to more than double between 2000 and 2040 (U.S. Administration on Aging, 2014). Concerns continue to mount regarding the ability to effectively provide health and social services for this growing population. In 2008, the Institute of Medicine of the National Academies reported that the healthcare workforce was not prepared to serve the needs of this growing number of older adults. One of its recommendations was to increase and improve recruitment and training efforts in geriatrics for disciplines such as medicine, nursing, and social work.

Similarly, a state-level report in West Virginia concluded that the long-term care workforce will be inadequate to meet the needs of the state's growing number of older adult residents and their families. This anticipated inadequacy stems from a smaller available pool of professionals who have less education and training and lower salaries than professionals in many other states (West Virginia Long-Term Care Partnership Workforce Working Group, 2010). This reality is compounded by the size of the elder population and the special issues confronting them. West Virginia has the second largest population of older persons in the nation; the state's older residents also have higher levels of poverty and disability than such individuals in other states. Almost 11% (compared to 10% nationally) of older West Virginians live below 100% of the federal poverty level, and 45% report having at least one disability, compared with 37% of older adults nationwide. Older West Virginians also have higher rates of chronic illness, such as heart disease (West Virginia Department of Health and Human Resources, 2012).

Given the crisis of an aging population and an inadequate workforce, the School of Social Work at West Virginia University initiated an action to improve the training of professionals in the state (particularly the long-term care workforce) by organizing an interdisciplinary workgroup of educators and professionals in the community to work collaboratively to attain the following objectives:

1. Evaluate the geriatric education needs of social workers (and related professionals with associate degrees and higher) in West Virginia.
2. Develop a gerontology practitioner certificate and curriculum.
3. Gain insight into means for retaining professionals in the field.

Addressing these three objectives confirmed the need for a continuing education (CE) gerontology practitioner's certificate program. Assessing the geriatric training needs of social work and other professionals, especially in aging, also provided insight and information on how to best recruit and retain professionals in gerontology in small towns and rural areas.

Literature Review

In 2011, the first "baby boomers" turned 65 years of age, initiating the much anticipated "silver tsunami." Aging adults are the world's fastest growing group, alerting social and health care providers to the increasing needs and requirements of this aging cohort. In addition to the global demographic changes occurring, the workforce servicing older adults also is aging, with more than 50% now 50 years of age or older (Frank et al., 2014). These two trends speak to the pressing need to address the aging community's mental, physical, and social needs, as well as the professional development of a small number of trained professionals (and a larger number of semi-skilled professionals) for working with older adults. Educating policymakers, program developers, community activists, mental and physical health care providers, and formal and informal caregiving specialists occurs both in the classroom and in the community. As such, developing a well-trained professional workforce that can meet the needs of aging citizens has been the goal of social workers for many years.

Supporting healthy aging through prevention, education, community resources, and long-term services was a major focus of the 2015 White House Conference on Aging (The White House Office of the Press Secretary, 2015). Awareness of the chronic health conditions and disparities in resources and services for older adults was a mobilizing call, as well as a recent national social work conference (National Association of Social Workers, 2015). The Affordable Care Act of 2010 included provisions for preventive health care for aging adults and racial minorities; however, most health care providers do not specialize in geriatrics or gerontology. Nonetheless, the Institute of Medicine of the National Academies (2008) expects that approximately 60% of adults age 65 and older will develop at least one chronic condition such as dementia, diabetes, heart disease, or musculoskeletal disorders. These chronic conditions most often result in the loss of independence, requiring a higher quantity and quality of care and demanding an educated, well-trained, and competent workforce. Training our current cohort of social workers and related professionals in the social and behavioral determinants of health of the aging thus must be accomplished through both traditional higher education and post-professional CE.

Geriatric Needs and Workforce Projections

Geriatric workforce shortages have been well documented and have been the focus of higher education initiatives for the past two decades, yet there continues to be a lack of both formal and informal training in gerontology (Teitelman & O'Neill, 2001). The Council on Social Work Education's (CSWE) Geriatric Social Work Initiative has developed competencies for social workers who provide services at all levels of service delivery (Social Work Leadership Institute, n.d.). Unfortunately, most schools of social work and health professions have not integrated the needs of aging adults across the curricula. As a result, many professionals are not trained to provide services to the current cohort of aging adults. In addition, according to the Council on Social Work Education (2011), only 5% of social work graduates specialize in aging, whereas data from a recent study indicate that less than

1% of nursing graduates have specialized training in aging and less than 3% of advanced nurse practitioners have their specialization in aging (Eldercare Workforce Alliance, 2014; Frank, 2015).

Workforce preparedness is partially contingent on the flexibility and versatility of continuing professional education. Tilleczek, Pong, and Caty (2005) reported that CE programs need to be convenient, short, and flexible and to provide opportunities for professional networking and support. Several studies have identified the efficacy of online and face-to-face workshops, summer institutes, and certificate programs in this regard (Congress, 2012; Congress, Englehardt, & Zeiders, 2007; Geron, Andrews, & Kuhn, 2005; Murphy-Southwick & McBride, 2006; Tumosa et al., 2012). Moreover, urban and rural social workers describe the utility and attractiveness of varied methods of delivering CE programs (Teitelman & O'Neill, 2001). For example, rural social workers report the desire for face-to-face professional development to alleviate the isolation that often accompanies rural social work practice (Murphy-Southwick & McBride, 2006). However, other professionals desire online, asynchronous learning opportunities that support their work and family schedules (Tilleczek et al., 2005).

Trends In Continuing Education and Professional Development

Previous research on the postprofessional, competency-based educational needs of mental and physical health service providers has identified some of the aging content training needs of the current work force cohort (Frank et al., 2014; Geron et al., 2005; Toner, Ferguson, & Davis Sokal, 2009). These content areas include training in physical health issues, including chronic conditions such as respiratory and heart disease, diabetes, musculoskeletal degeneration, pain related disorders, and declining mobility. Education related to mental health issues facing aging populations include depression and anxiety; suicide; bereavement; cognitive and neurodegenerative disorders; and substance abuse involving alcohol, prescription medications, and illegal drugs (Toner et al., 2009). There are issues of rising medical costs, concerns about being underinsured, and a lack of accessibility to healthcare facilities. Furthermore, many older adults experience insecure or inadequate housing, poor nutrition, social isolation, lack of social supports, and limited caregiving alternatives.

Recent studies have identified models of training programs and methods of delivery that meet the needs of postgraduate professionals (Congress, 2012; Tumosa et al., 2012). Face-to-face pedagogical models were identified as particularly helpful for rural workers who frequently find themselves working alone, in isolation, and often crossing traditional professional boundaries and "wearing multiple hats" to serve the needs of rural community members (Murphy-Southwick & McBride, 2006). Methods of delivery include online synchronous and asynchronous courses, webinars, home study courses—especially those that are inexpensive and short in duration. Workshops, institutes, and conferences that allow for interdisciplinary dialogue also are welcome.

Competency-based training that is easily transferrable to practice settings, relevant to community based needs assessment, and focused on skill development also are key components identified by previous evaluations (Geron et al., 2005). As part of the National Center for Gerontological Social Work Education, CSWE outlined core competencies within competency domains of gerontology, cultural competence, person-centered care, and participant-direction. Adult professional learners welcome the opportunity to learn new material and to share and integrate their own experiences into practice-relevant content and skill-based strategies. Building on practice skills, professional development and CE must be dynamic, experiential, and interactive (Tumosa et al., 2012).

Finally, with tightening budgets and increased demand for developing a trained workforce, individuals and agencies are looking for the most cost-effective means of developing skills and acquiring new knowledge. Continuing education via web-based delivery, weekend institutes, workshops, and conferences provides the answer to several needs: (a) how to reach the largest number of professionals working with older adults; (b) how to provide cost-effective professional development that meets a transferability litmus test; and (c) how to offer incentives for increasing one's expertise, meeting licensure requirements, and improving recruitment and retention of service providers. This study sought to assess the need to create one such program and evaluate its outcomes.

Methods

To conduct the needs assessment, the School of Social Work began by gathering an interdisciplinary, statewide workgroup. Members represented social work, nursing, counseling, and pastoral care from settings such as higher education, private practice, community-based agencies, home care providers, hospices, and long-term care settings, and they were selected based on their varied professional training and experience, geographic area of practice, and interest in gerontology education. (Two authors of this article co-chaired the group.) The workgroup members were located across the state, so meetings utilizing conference call technology (for some of the more remote participants) were held in order to begin the development of a survey to assess the aging education needs of social workers and related professionals, as well as inquire about the best ways to attract and retain quality workers in the field. Participants identified key survey questions and devised a sampling and data collection plan. Professionals targeted for the survey included counselors, nurses, nursing home administrators, pharmacists, social workers, family caregivers, educators, and professionals in the faith community. Finalized and then approved by the university's Institutional Review Board, the survey was administered online using a survey development service. Participants were recruited to complete the online survey through listservs and e-mail contacts.

Results

Survey

The survey developed by the workgroup consisted of 26 items, the majority of which were closed-ended. Questions focused on attitudes toward a gerontology certificate program, including whether respondents would be interested in enrolling, what they would expect to gain from the program, topic areas that should be included, training format preferences (including online offerings), and expectations regarding cost. Background inquiries also were made related to the geographic area in which respondents lived and worked, experience in the field of aging, current role and work setting, educational background, discipline, and licensure. A few questions also solicited information about what led respondents to the field of gerontology practice and what factors would likely keep them in the field. The responses to closed-ended questions were analyzed using descriptive statistics. An open-ended question asked respondents if they had additional comments that would help us better understand the need and/or curriculum for a gerontology practitioner certificate. The responses to this question, as well as those that allowed respondents to contribute "other" responses than those listed, or expand on answers to closed-ended questions, were analyzed using a basic analysis of themes. In this analysis, answers were reviewed, patterns were identified, and themes were developed and applied to the data.

Respondents

Invitations to participate in the survey were e-mailed to several listservs and to contacts of the workgroup. A total of 391 individuals completed the survey. Percentages are presented followed by a sample size for each question, as not all participants completed every question. The majority of respondents who identified a discipline in terms of education were trained as social workers (46%, $n = 164$), followed by nurses and speech pathologists (each 16%, $n = 57$). Professionals with backgrounds in education, counseling, sociology, and psychology each represented about 3% of the respondents. Most had earned a bachelor's (27%, $n = 97$) or master's (56%, $n = 195$) degree in their identified discipline, and more than 85% also held a professional license. In terms of formal geriatric training, 43% ($n = 153$) identified CE offerings as the primary or sole source. Thirty-three percent ($n = 118$) indicated that they had no formal training in aging or geriatrics.

Looking at the workplaces of the respondents, almost 60% ($n = 208$) reported that their primary place of employment serves a 50% or higher rate of older clients, with 26% ($n = 93$) of workplaces reported as almost exclusively serving older adults, more than 90%. Almost 40% ($n = 145$) worked in health care organizations such as hospice, hospital, nursing home, dialysis, physician office, or home health care. Fourteen percent ($n = 49$) worked for the state-level Department of Health and Human Services. Regarding professional roles represented, the majority (44%, $n = 159$) were in direct/clinical practice, followed by supervisors and administrators (19%, $n = 71$). Respondents were very diverse in terms of the number of years they had been employed in geriatric services, from less than 1 to more than 30 years in the field. Finally, survey respondents either lived or worked in 36 out of 55 counties in West Virginia, as well as the bordering states of Pennsylvania, Ohio, Kentucky, and Virginia.

Interest in the Gerontology Practitioner Certificate and Training Needs

The majority of questions in the survey sought to determine respondents' levels of interest in a gerontology practitioner certificate program and the desired curriculum for such a course of study. Within the survey, a curriculum structure—based on a previous CE aging certificate offered a decade earlier by another department in the university—was adapted by the workgroup and presented as a possible educational program. The majority (77%, $n = 300$) of respondents expressed some interest in enrolling in the certificate program, as presented, within the next 2 years. More than 70% selected increased knowledge ($n = 254$) and competence ($n = 242$) as major reasons for enrolling. In addition, personal satisfaction and growth (67%, $n = 221$), as well as meeting professional licensure requirements (60%, $n = 195$), were selected as reasons to enroll.

A variety of answers were stated as reasons that respondents would not enroll in the program. The top ranking responses included personal cost (14%, $n = 27$), amount of time to complete the certificate (14%, $n = 27$), and lack of perceived career benefit (15%, $n = 28$). Of those who were not interested in enrolling, some (19%, $n = 37$) stated that they would consider enrolling if CE events were offered near them, or if a portion of the required hours were offered online (21%, $n = 40$). Similarly, 85% of all respondents ($n = 312$) said that they would be likely or very likely to access certificate training online regardless of whether they enrolled in the program.

Respondents also were asked to provide additional comments regarding the need for the development of a gerontology practitioner certificate. Fifty-three responses were provided, and the comments were diverse, including specific information about respondents' current work with older adults and future educational goals. An overwhelming theme, mentioned by 20 respondents, stated a strong commitment to meeting the needs of older adults. This commitment was evident in the following comments:

- I would LOVE the opportunity to learn more and pass the information along to the many older residents in our community to help to improve the quality of life for these individuals.
- A curriculum is very much needed for our workers to understand the population that we are dealing with, and the need is urgent.
- The population of the country is aging, so no matter the discipline, this is an area in which we all need to become more competent.
- The population warrants that we improve and expand our skill sets. We are an aging population in an aging state, surrounded by aging states in an aging world.

Respondents were asked to select a variety of subject areas in which they wanted or felt they needed more training. Almost half selected clients' cognitive changes ($n = 181$), dementia ($n = 171$), and end-of-life issues ($n = 177$). More than 30% also were interested in legal issues ($n = 118$) and health and social policies and programs ($n = 127$). Respondents noted that they currently meet their CE needs primarily through employer-based trainings (33%, $n = 121$). More than 20% of the respondents also reported attendance at the annual National Association of Social Workers state conference ($n = 81$) and the School's Summer Institute on Aging ($n = 77$) and similar school-sponsored workshops ($n = 80$).

Online training was indicated as a preferred training method, with 69% ($n = 251$) noting this as a format that would be most beneficial for attaining CE. A mixture of lecture and experiential-style training was preferred (44%, $n = 162$). Several locations were noted as those to which respondents would be willing to travel for trainings, with two larger cities in the state each reflecting the preference of more than 39% ($n = 141, 161$) of respondents. In terms of paying for training, many (32%, $n = 117$) were not sure how much they currently pay for 1 hour of CE, whereas more than 38% ($n = 141$) believed they paid less than $15 per hour. About the same number of respondents indicated that they would pay less than $15 per hour for an online training.

Retention of Professionals in the Field

An additional (but smaller) objective of the survey was to gain insight into the retention of professionals in the field. When asked what led them to work in gerontology, many noted a job opportunity (57%, $n = 201$), as well as personal and family experiences (29%, $n = 101$). Forty-one respondents specified an "other" factor that drew them to the field, and two main themes emerged from these responses. Seventeen mentioned having exposure to older adults in their professional fields, such as audiology, health care, counseling, domestic violence, and massage therapy. Twelve respondents mentioned that they always "enjoyed" or "loved" this population or had an interest or passion for working with elders. Similarly, a follow-up question asked the respondents to expand on the answers they gave to this question. Forty-five responses fell under three main themes. The "love" of the population was again noted, with 10 respondents expressing this sentiment and citing elders as sources of knowledge and great inspiration. Twenty-four described a professional or educational background that led them to the field. Of interest, nine respondents specifically mentioned personal experiences with grandparents or other older relatives as driving forces for their entry into the field.

In response to what factors would keep them in the field, increased opportunity for career growth ($n = 165$) and increased salary and benefits ($n = 140$) were selected by more than 40% of respondents. An increased opportunity for leadership in the field was chosen by 28% ($n = 98$). An additional theme that emerged reflected a recognition of the growing number of older adults, the need to increase training on their behalf, and a genuine love for the population. For example,

- I feel as the older population increases there will be an increased demand and opportunity to work with older people. I feel it is important to have people that have had specific training in this area to work with them.
- No motivation is needed. I love the population, and I intend to continue working with them, regardless of pay-rate or CE.
- I love what I do and just want to keep doing it. Beyond the CE requirement for licensure, I enjoy obtaining new information that will help me and those I serve.

Resulting Program and Follow-Up

The Gerontology Practitioner Certificate (GPC) was formally launched in June 2013. The curriculum for the program requires participants to complete 100 clock hours of CE over the course of 4 years in a variety of content and skill areas related to gerontology. Specifically, GPC enrollees must complete at least 6 hours in each of the content areas of Physiological Processes and Health in Older Adults, Psychosocial Processes and Mental Health in Older Adults, Social Policy and Aging, Aspects of Rural Aging, and Aging and Ethics, as well as a minimum of 6 hours in the skill areas of Communication, Assessment, Counseling/Interviewing, Case Management, and Management. To provide flexibility and specialization for participants, the remaining 40 hours may be fulfilled in any of the designated content and skill areas. A minimum of 30 hours must be earned by participating in CE events sponsored by the West Virginia University School of Social Work.

The content and skill areas for the GPC were developed by the interdisciplinary workgroup based on the data provided from the needs assessment survey. To make face-to-face programming more accessible to a rural statewide audience and to address survey respondents' concerns that there be enough face-to-face programs nearby or online, the GPC is designed so that both participants and outside CE providers can seek GPC approval for programming. This resulted in 16 outside training entities receiving approval for 113 workshops and conferences, from June 2013 to October 2015. Moreover, many of these trainings are purposefully interdisciplinary, increasing participants' interactions with persons from a variety of backgrounds and professional expertise. To further address the survey respondents' concerns of accessibility, an additional means of training was provided through the five 6-hour online CE courses developed at the School of Social Work for this program. In addition, an outside provider, the WV Alzheimer's Association, offered a 34 clock hour online Dementia Care Training Course.

The interdisciplinary workgroup that initially developed the structure and the curriculum for the GPC evolved into a monitoring group, reviewing and approving requests for workshop and conference approvals, by both GPC participants and outside CE providers. This function has proved critical to the growth and accessibility of the GPC program, as these gerontology education partners are able to provide programming in topic areas and at locales that the School of Social Work is not able to easily serve, expanding the accessibility and diversity of educational opportunities for GPC participants.

As of April 30, 2016, there were 66 people enrolled in the GPC program: 30 applied in 2013, 17 in 2014, 18 in 2015, and one thus far in 2016. The demographics of the enrollees are very similar to those of the respondents of the needs assessment survey. More than half of the participants (55%, $n = 36$) are licensed social workers, and the next largest professional affiliation is nurses (12%, $n = 8$). Enrollment by persons without a professional affiliation is currently at 23% ($n = 15$) and 26% ($n = 17$) of the participants identify as a current or former family caregiver. Ninety-three of the participants in the program reside in West Virginia, and 7% live in Pennsylvania, Ohio, Maryland, or North Carolina.

The majority of participants (93%, $n = 61$) have a college education; 38% ($n = 25$) have a bachelor's degree, 50% ($n = 33$) have a master's, and 5%

(n = 3) have a doctorate. People enrolled in the GPC report a wide (but fairly even) distribution of gerontology-related work experience. Of the 39 participants who indicated their years of experience, 2% (n = 1) have 1 year of experience or less, 18% (n = 7) have 2 to 5 years of experience, 28% (n = 11) have 6 to 10 years of experience, 21% (n = 8) have 11 to 20 years; and 26% (n = 10) have more than 20 years of experience. Regarding the workplaces of the participants, almost 77% (n = 51) reported that their place of employment serves primarily older adult clients.

Discussion

The survey provides new knowledge for determining the need for a gerontology practitioner certificate program. Providing low-cost and web-based opportunities encourages a majority of professionals to participate in certificate trainings. Also, reviewing offerings at state conferences for compliance with certificate credit is proactive in extending education and recruitment opportunities.

Regardless of overall program successes, there are limitations to be noted as well. As in most efforts to assess interest and develop new programs, there are ways to grow and improve. The first noted limitation is survey bias in terms of the disciplines and backgrounds of the participants. Despite enlisting a multidisciplinary workgroup, and sending announcements out on a variety of professional listservs, social workers represent the overwhelming majority of respondents. Special efforts were made to attract disciplines that were underrepresented, including nursing and speech, occupational, and physical therapy. Such additional recruitment did appear to attract nurses, speech pathologists, and audiologists. One cohort that emerged across disciplines was professionals who currently were, or had previously been, family caregivers themselves.

Another limitation was the mode of recruitment and of program delivery. Although online survey recruitment and surveys have become commonplace, this modality may have eliminated the opinions of a large group of people who were not on listservs or who did not wish to complete an online survey.

Despite these limitations, the workgroup believed that delivering the GPC is a valuable endeavor to better prepare professionals in the field of geriatrics. Enrollment numbers in just this one CE gerontology program confirm the need as well. All states are experiencing increasing numbers of older adults and may be poorly prepared to meet the need for geriatric education at the undergraduate, graduate, and postgraduate (CE) levels. Many professionals come to geriatrics postgraduation and often have very little formal instruction on the unique issues of this client population. There is consequently an increasing demand for professionals specifically trained in geriatric services who will remain in this growing field of practice.

Implications

Launching the GPC has not been without its challenges, and other programs in higher education can learn from this process of gathering a workgroup, developing a needs assessment, conducting a survey, and implementing a program in response to identified needs. To begin, schools should carefully evaluate staff resources to execute such a program, should an assessment determine feasibility and a need. In this program, the lack of administrative capacity to fully implement the program was the biggest and most troublesome issue. In June 2013, the staff of the School of Social Work Professional & Community Education Program office consisted of a full-time coordinator, a 0.5 FTE secretary, and a 20-hr-per-week graduate assistant. Although the needs assessment indicated a demand for the program, staff underestimated the time that would be needed to adequately administer the program and was not well prepared to respond to the mounting enrollment requests of prospective participants. The processing of new applications, review of participants' and outside educational entities' requests for GPC approval, tracking of participants' progress, and publicity and outreach requisites quickly became too much for the small staff to adequately manage. Therefore, in October 2013, a graduate student position was opened at 15 hours per week to help manage the ongoing and day-to-day running of the CE certificate programs, and this addition of an extra staff person continues to be necessary to effectively manage enrollment and monitor the day-to-day duties associated with the GPC.

The composition of and process for working with a workgroup also were key considerations, especially when its role evolved from program development to monitoring. Several people left the group after the GPC was launched, and subsequent discussions revealed that the time-limited role (of assessing needs and developing curricula) were their main interests. The ongoing role of monitoring was not as appealing. Nevertheless, most of the original interdisciplinary workgroup remained involved. However, clearer expectations of workgroup members was an important finding.

Other schools seeking to develop a CE program in gerontology should also consider factors such as flexibility, accessibility, and affordability. One of the strengths of the GPC program proved to be its flexibility in allowing participants to focus their personal and professional development on gerontology content and skill areas that were most meaningful to them. This strength, however, was also one of the challenges in the GPC design. No two participants completing the GPC had the exact same educational experience, which made evaluation of the program difficult. Offering content online (or face-to-face in areas that were convenient for participants) and approving the trainings of partner organizations increased accessibility. The issue of fees and affordability, of course, should be a central consideration as well.

Initiatives of the John A. Hartford Foundation have provided many tools and programs for the infusion of geriatric content into undergraduate and graduate social work curricula, as well as opportunities for students to receive specialized course and field training in serving older adults (Hooyman, 2009). Surveys and their results, similar to the needs assessment conducted by the GPC program at West Virginia University, also can help to inform for-credit social work education in this critical area.

Conclusion

The silver tsunami of baby boomers is marching on. The geriatric work-force also is aging, as are older adults who rely on their services. Opportunities for ongoing education and networking can be delivered in a variety of ways, but a critical factor is that of making offerings available to meet the need and context of those likely to enroll (Congress et al., 2007). Regardless of setting, urban and rural social workers seek CE for licensure, as well as professional growth (Teitelman & O'Neill, 2001), hence the CE option is a propitious one to pursue. In this regard, we should follow the advice of Lao-Tzu: "Deal with it before it happens. Set things in order before there is confusion."

Acknowledgments

We thank the WV Partnership in Elder Living, WV Community Voices, Inc., and the Claude W. Benedum Foundation for their support of this project. The project would also not have been possible without the work of our workgroup members: Jeanie Brenneman, Nancy Daugherty, Sherry Kuhl, Judith Wilkinson, Phillip Donnelly, Deloris Wilder, Gail Mason, Betty Maxwell, Kandi Taylor, and Susie Layne.

References

Administration on Aging. (2014). *A profile of older Americans: 2014*. Washington, DC: United States Department of Health and Human Services, Administration on Aging, Administration for Community Living. Retrieved from http://www.aoa.gov/Aging_Statistics/Profile/2014/docs/2014-Profile.pdf

Congress, E. P. (2012). Guest editorial continuing education: Lifelong learning for social work practitioners and educators. *Journal of Social Work Education, 48*(3), 397–401. doi:10.5175/JSWE.2012.201200085

Congress, E., Englehardt, J., & Zeiders, A. (2007, October). *Evidence-based continuing education and professional development*. Paper presented at the Council on Social Work Education Annual Program Meeting, San Francisco, CA.

Council on Social Work Education. (2011). 2009 Statistics on social work education in the United States. Retrieved from http://www.cswe.org/CentersInitiatives/DataStatistics/ProgramData/47673.aspx

Eldercare Workforce Alliance. (2014). *Geriatrics workforce shortage: A looming crisis for our families*. Retrieved from http://www.eldercareworkforce.org/research/issue-briefs/research: geriatrics-workforce-shortage-a-looming-crisis-for-our-families/

Frank, J. C. (2015). A missing piece in the infrastructure to promote healthy aging programs: Education and work force development. *Frontiers in Public Health, 2*(287), 1–3. doi:10.3389/fpubh.2014.00287

Frank, J. C., Altpeter, M., Damron-Rodriguez, J., Driggers, J., Lachenmayr, S., Manning, C., … Robinson, P. (2014). Preparing the workforce for healthy aging programs: The skills for healthy aging resources and programs (SHARP) model. *Health Education and Behavior, 41*(Suppl. 1), 19S–26S. doi:10.1177/1090198114543007

Geron, S. M., Andrews, C., & Kuhn, K. (2005). Infusing aging skills into the social work practice community: A new look at strategies for continuing professional education. *Families in Society: The Journal of Contemporary Social Services, 86*(3), 431–440. doi:10.1606/1044-3894.3442

Hooyman, N. R. (2009). *Transforming social work education: The first decade of the Hartford geriatric social work initiative*. Alexandria, VA: Council on Social Work Education.

Institute of Medicine of the National Academies. (2008, April 11). *Retooling for an aging America: Building the health care workforce*. Washington, DC: National Academies Press.

Murphy-Southwick, C., & McBride, M. (2006). Geriatric education across 94 million acres: Adapting conference programming in a rural state. *Gerontology & Geriatrics Education, 26*(4), 25–36. doi:10.1300/J021v26n04_03

National Association of Social Workers. (2015). NASW comments to the White House Conference on Aging. Retrieved from http://www.socialworkers.org/practice/aging/whcoa2015comments.asp

Social Work Leadership Institute. (n.d.). *Geriatric Social Work Competency Scale II with Life Long Leadership Skills*. Retrieved from http://www.cswe.org/File.aspx?id=25445

Teitelman, J. L., & O'Neill, P. (2001). Adult development and aging: A model continuing education course for practicing social workers. *Journal of Gerontological Social Work, 35*(4), 57–67. doi:10.1300/J083v35n04_05

Tilleczek, K., Pong, R., & Caty, S. (2005). Innovations and issues in the delivery of continuing education to nurse practitioners in rural and northern communities. *Canadian Journal of Nursing Research, 37*(1), 147–162.

Toner, J. A., Ferguson, D. K., & Davis Sokal, R. (2009). Continuing interprofessional education in geriatrics and gerontology in medically underserved areas. *Journal of Continuing Education in the Health Professions, 29*(3), 157–160. doi:10.1002/chp.20029

Tumosa, N., Horvath, K. J., Huh, T., Livote, E., Howe, J. L., Jones, L. I., & Kramer, B. J. (2012). Health care workforce development in rural America: When geriatrics expertise is 100 miles away. *Gerontology & Geriatrics Education, 33*, 133–151. doi:10.1080/02701960.2012.661812

West Virginia Department of Health and Human Resources. (2012, June 6). *Older West Virginians: Health highlights*. Retrieved from http://www.wvdhhr.org/bph/hsc/statserv/Pub.asp?ID=167

West Virginia Long-Term Care Partnership Workforce Working Group. (2010). *Workforce Working Group: Final report and recommendations*. Retrieved from:http://www.wvpel.org/downloads/Summit2010/Workforce%20Overview%20and%20Recom mendations.pdf

The White House Office of the Press Secretary. (2015). *The White House Conference on Aging: Empowering all Americans as we age* (Fact sheet). Retrieved from https://www.whitehouse.gov/the-press-office/2015/07/13/fact-sheet-white-house-conference-aging

Connecting Social Work and Activism in the Arts Through Continuing Professional Education

Kathryn Rawdon and David Moxley

ABSTRACT

The authors place a continuing education conference devoted to linking the arts, social practice, and social work within the context of a movement to advance arts activism. They illustrate how social workers, artists, and community arts activists can collaborate in building public awareness about serious social issues, creating alternative explanations of the causes of those issues, and producing opportunity structures for people experiencing social marginalization. By connecting arts activism and social work through the use of common values pertaining to social justice, social workers can engage the arts as a vehicle for social betterment.

Introduction

Social workers can benefit from their involvement in the arts as a way of advancing practice, particularly with people who face numerous social challenges resulting in their marginalization. Increasingly, artists are engaged in forms of social activism, including the creation of opportunities for people who do not readily fit into normative structures, the use of arts in raising public consciousness of social issues, and the advancement of new conceptions of how society can be more inclusive.

Art is evolving from forms of expression, under the control of elites, into more populist ones found in raw art [art brut], folk, vernacular, and naïve forms. Those diverse populist forms share their capacity for enabling people who are not necessarily trained artists to express perspectives on their lived experience in community life or in society at large. These populist forms of outsider art find the most relevance when people express their voice, oftentimes involving a critique of societal arrangements (Johnson, 2010).

Artists contribute to a broader context that we refer to as *social practice* in this article. Social practice involves the actions that individuals and groups take to advance social betterment in society. Such practice may include scientists, humanists, ecologists, social scientists, and citizens who share in efforts to advocate progressive improvements in society. Artists, in particular, are unique in social practice, as their interpretative approaches to representation and self-expression can create new meanings that one could come to assign to social issues that he or she does not readily understand or experience (Eisner, 2008). Interpreters of societal conditions may be one of the most important roles that artists as activists play in society. They can collaborate with other social practitioners in advancing perspectives about social conditions, engaging in protest, and organizing action to address societal issues and injustice (Campana, 2011).

Arts activism also can foster the development of social infrastructure consistent with the aims of social work. The arts lend themselves to the formation of social and mutual support for people who experience marginalization (Moxley, 2013). Reaching people who may not otherwise become involved in the arts, arts programs and studios appear to be accelerating in diverse social problem domains including homelessness, serious mental illness, dementia, cancer, other serious physical illnesses, and developmental disabilities. Such programs do not incorporate therapy through the arts but focus on the development of individuals as practicing and productive artists. The arts also can facilitate the formation of identities for people experiencing oppression or marginalization (Moxley, 2014). Studios themselves offer creative environments in which people can explore artful self-expression regarding the conditions under which they live.

By offering opportunities that support people's representations of the issues they face in their daily lives, as well as the conditions in which they exist, these artists can express their identities, including the degradation they may experience in society. Such critical portrayals can be found in vernacular, raw art, or naïve forms of artistic self-expression. Not only does such art offer an avenue of self-expression, even catharsis, for those experiencing marginalization, but such depictions can create cohesion among persons sharing a social reality (Elmendorff, 2009). Studios, galleries, and arts education events can strengthen group life among their participants, furthering the aims of social work by offering people experiencing marginalization a community in which they can form social attachments, form identities, and emerge as self-taught artists. Such artists play off their own experience, using self-expression to communicate a perspective on social conditions, including degrading ones that may be found in art brut or other forms of vernacular expression.

Continuing education programs in social work can build bridges among activist artists involved in social practice, arts advocates, and social work professionals. Indeed, one of the important functions of continuing education in social work is to convene social workers so they can consider new avenues of practice. Inclusion of the arts is one of these innovations. In this spirit, the continuing education program at the University of Oklahoma

Anne and Henry Zarrow School of Social Work has focused on inclusion of the arts as an important element of its strategy for augmenting innovation in social work practice within the state of Oklahoma. In this article, we examine a 2015 Arts and Social Practice Conference in which social workers came together with artists, arts activists, and human service professionals to consider how the arts can facilitate opportunities for people whose marginalization can easily segregate them from existing opportunity structures within communities. The conference was designed to reach multiple groups of participants (social work, health and human services, and the arts), including practitioners, administrators, and policymakers.

The Program for Continuing Education in Social Work

Initiated 4 years ago, the Program for Continuing Education in Social Work at the University of Oklahoma School of Social Work developed its profile of continuing education options strategically. Prior to the initiation of this program, the school had offered one major social work conference a year. However, by 2015, the program offered more than 95 continuing educational events, making available 300 potential continuing education credits to 800 participants. Since its founding 4 years ago, this program has provided continuing education to 2,100 social workers.

The events themselves are quite diverse, involving weekly seminars and workshops, quarterly conferences, full-day symposia, and web-based options including a monthly ongoing book club in the human services. Experimenting with other media to support continuing education, the program has sponsored a professional development certificate in adult learning and aging, and a sequence of offerings in other substantive areas of social work practice. More recent content particularly facilitates the preparation of social workers for licensure renewal.

The program's curriculum model incorporates adult learning principles. It recognizes the relevant practice experiences that social workers and other human service professionals bring to continuing education sessions. There are five objectives of the continuing education program: (a) offering participants an ongoing venue for fulfilling their continuing education needs through adult education, (b) providing contexts in which participants can increase their insight into social work practice through collaborative learning among those attending sessions, (c) augmenting innovative perspectives on social work practice, (d) diversifying learning methods and strategies so participants can achieve their own professional development learning goals, and (e) using diverse formats to foster easy access to continuing education.

The arts came into play within the program during the early part of 2015. In partnership with the school's Knee Center for Strong Families, the program began the process of strengthening the linkage between social work and the arts via continuing education. This link was an interest of the benefactor of the Knee Center, Ruth Knee, a social work pioneer, and within the state of Oklahoma, where a strong interest in public health also extends to the arts and social work. Sharing an interest in the arts, we framed an initial conference to advance the linkage; further intellectual engagement of the arts with social practice; convene social workers, human service professionals, artists, and other social practitioners to consider the theory and practice of the arts in social practice; and examine local exemplars that connect the arts and social practice. The first author coordinated this effort and piloted an initial conference to assess the interest in the arts and social practice among both practitioners in the human services and the arts.

The Arts and Human Development

The arts likely came about early in human evolution as a means for strengthening group cohesion among human beings. Individuals engaged in the arts because such expression created the group identity so integral to self-protection and survival in uncertain environments (Boylan, 2008). The diversity in ways of expressing group life (through various art forms) created numerous avenues for reinforcing group life, such as visual representation, and music. For some, such as Australian Aboriginal people, art forms linked artistic expression to practical applications found in how song could create cognitive maps through which group members could navigate seemingly hostile terrain.

The fusion of the arts and practical use enabled humans to create technology that not only served particular purposes but also offered a symbolic representation of group life, thereby reinforcing group membership and identity (Zeisel, 2004). Likely paralleling the growth of the human brain, the emergence of symbolism in art took on even more influence in human groups, as artists, lay or professional, could capture through symbols the group's beliefs about the cosmos, the world, and local geographies, etching these in pottery, tools, and even weapons. The evolution of symbolism as an art form itself freed human beings solely from literal representation of objects to the interpretation of alternate realities, thereby producing meaning that could inspire human action (Allen, 1995).

As an act of making meaning, representation through interpretation would come to politicize art as human expression. Interpretation as symbol making deepened the possibilities of artful representation and, in many cases, released the artist from prior strictures of representation so the artist could serve as critic of society, rather than merely as a bard, affirming existing social structures (Carey, 2006; Escobar, 1994). The artist as critic anticipates the emergence of artists as dissidents who produce alternative views of reality as portraits of what could be, or what should not be, in terms of a criticism of situations that may be degrading the existence of human beings (Belfiore & Bennett, 2008). Ultimately, artists control aesthetics, creating ways of expressing their own emotions or influencing the emotions of others who use, engage, or collect artful products.

Although discussing the role of the arts in business, particularly its influence on creative engagement, Austen (2010) apprised us of how the arts can fuse both cognition and emotion. For Austen, the cognitive-emotions, like wonder, can move artists and consumers of the arts from the now to the future. The arts can facilitate anticipation of what can be, whether such representations may be negative or positive, dystopian or utopian, views of the future. The integral connection of the arts and human development suggests for the authors the possibility that people can enact, use, and engage the arts as a means for expanding their horizons, for learning about experiences they may initially find alien, or for crafting possibilities for the expansion of human awareness and insight (Boeck, Moxley, & Wachter, 2011).

Social practice in the arts affirms the critical as an essential perspective in taking action for social betterment in society. The alignment of social work with the arts harnesses the possibilities of social criticism as a means for motivating and structuring social action. Collaboration among social workers and artists can open up vistas neither group may be able to produce on their own (Brandt, 2008). Creative synergies among those in the helping professions and those who represent society through the arts can define new options for human development across the life course, both in particular situations and in society as a whole (Feen-Calligan, Washington, & Moxley, 2009). Artists serve to augment information in society, which more normative actors may eschew in the name of stability. One strategy for increasing information can occur when artists memorialize events to increase societal awareness of injustice. (Harvey, 1996; Junge, 1999; Kaminsky, 1984; Watkins & Shulman, 2008). Artists can use information embedded in their representations to encourage dissent (Sunstein, 2003; Zinn, 2003). A resulting expansion of human awareness, whether this occurs at individual, group, or higher order social systems, contributes considerably to the advancement of human development (Eisner, 2004). Compared to science, the arts represent a different way of knowing and acting (Eisner, 1981), although increasingly there are efforts to integrate the arts and science, particularly in the production of innovative products through which people meet their needs, especially for survival in difficult situations (Edwards, 2010a, 2010b).

Local Exemplars Inspiring Continuing Education in the Arts and Social Work

The three examples we offer next are a subset of a number of different community-based efforts operating in Oklahoma City. The city itself is within the top 10 arts markets in the United States, but even with considerable arts assets, the availability of community-based arts options for marginalized and/or underserved populations is quite limited.

The three examples reflect the qualities of community-based arts efforts that form a common base of action, melding the arts and social practice: (a) accessibility of art making to members of those populations who would normally be unable to access the arts, arts production, or arts education; (b) development of participants as artists, using the key features of the studio, whether in the visual arts or music education; (c) creating productive interactions and sustained relationships among emerging and practicing artists, as well as arts entrepreneurs and community leaders; (d) involvement of emerging artists with the public via exhibits, educational forums, or performances; (e) interactions of the arts with social action as a means of advancing public understanding of the social issues that often serve as the foci of participants' art self-expression; and (f) melding of the artistic production of participants with opportunities for their involvement in entrepreneurship. These three examples share their commitment to facilitating the development of emerging artists whose stories may become the themes of their art as they express them oftentimes through alternative methods of outsider art brut, vernacular, folk, or naïve forms of self-expression. By interrogating these three examples, we found considerable relevance for social workers when one focused on understanding the social purpose of community-based arts as involving more than bringing people together to produce art.

So, for us, these three examples offered a way of conceptualizing the development of the Arts and Social Practice Conference. This conference would come to serve as a vehicle for bringing together artists, arts educators, social workers, and human service professionals to consider how the arts can become a strategy for advancing social change.

Engaging Homeless People as Emerging Artists Through Fresh Start Studio

The Fresh stART studio began as a pilot program at the WestTown Day Shelter in April 2008, sponsored by the Homeless Alliance of Oklahoma City. The inspiration for its founding was the documentary film *Art from the Streets*, which profiles participants in a successful community arts program in Austin, Texas (http://www.artfromthestreets.org). The Fresh stART studio is the only program of its kind in the Oklahoma City metro area, offering studio space and art-making materials to adults who are currently or formerly homeless.

The studio provides quality arts instruction and promotes the work of studio artists through art shows and gallery exhibits. Fresh stART artists have shown artwork in 10 public venues, partnering with other nonprofit organizations such as the Oklahoma Chapter of the National Alliance on Mental Illness, Thunderbird Clubhouse, and Historic Capitol Hill. Such exhibits provide Fresh stART artists with income from sales of prints and original works. Through the exhibits, and through the very competent artwork of the emerging artists of Fresh stART, those visiting the exhibits come to see the social factors influencing homelessness.

The founders of Fresh stART recognized the value of offering a visual arts program as a means of helping people experiencing homelessness to combat the hardships they faced in their daily lives. The artists who participate in the Fresh stART studio, now more than 100, express feelings of accomplishment, increased self-esteem and self-worth, and release of anger and frustration through their involvement in art making. Studio participants are also able to bond with a community of artists from similar circumstances, interact with practicing artists who make a livelihood through the arts, and engage mentors who nurture their artistic spirit.

Engaging Girls With Limited Access to the Arts Through the Oklahoma City Girls Art School

The Oklahoma City Girls Art School seeks to empower girls from underserved communities to become successful in life by learning about the arts, developing their talents as emerging artists, and becoming members of an intentional community of artists. This alternative school stands outside of the public school system and offers high-quality visual arts training, introducing girls to successful female artists in the community, and giving the girls an opportunity to experience how the arts contribute to community life. The ultimate goal of the Oklahoma City Girls Art School is to inspire a love of the arts among emerging artists and to foster their appreciation of a creative discipline, enabling them to acquire personal assets such as confidence, imagination, tolerance, and social skills—particularly those involving teamwork and collaboration.

For social work, the school represents the development of an alternative community institution dedicated to helping girls obtain tangible skills in the areas of academic performance, career development, creativity, and social interaction. The curriculum assists the girls not only to develop as emerging artists but also to become aware of the arts as a vital aspect of society and as essential to advancing creative engagement in the world. Indeed, the curriculum folds those aims together so students can appreciate the essential value of creativity in social action. To effect such a connection, the girls engage in arts community service in which they can make contributions to community life through murals, arts events, and exhibits.

Restoring Music Education in High-Need Communities Through Bring Back the Music

Founded in 2010 by a creative jazz educator, Bring Back the Music provides access to quality and high-expectation performing arts education for youth from low-income communities. The organization began as an after-school venture, but it has since taken its program and curriculum into public schools, where music programs have suffered due to budget cuts. The organization partners with local elementary and middle schools to advance music education; facilitate the development of participants as practicing musicians; and offer opportunities for youth to develop social skills, creativity, and career awareness through music education.

Students who participate in the program learn to play instruments, receive vocal training, and learn choreography and music theory from experienced music professionals and educators. The curriculum also introduces students to music production software and hardware. They have an opportunity to write and record their own music, produce hip-hop using LogicPro, and perform their own work live before real audiences.

Although all participating youth can build their profiles, expand their experiences, and strengthen their portfolios in music as a primary vocation or career focus, the organization recognizes a potential of the arts for helping young people deepen their personal, social, and cultural qualities as effective individuals transitioning into adulthood. Thus, Bring Back the Music is developmental in its orientation to social action.

Implications of the Exemplars for Linking Social Work and the Arts

The three exemplars serve as models of what can occur when social innovators engage in organizing the arts for the purpose of advancing the development of people who may not see themselves as artists or creative individuals. The involvement of social workers as facilitators of such human development through the arts suggests a meaningful but perhaps emergent locus of practice. However, it is within this domain that social workers, partnering with social practitioners, can create arts options within communities diminished by socioeconomic inequality. Creating arts-based opportunity structures can serve as a means of realizing core social work values such as respect for the social attachments of people who experience marginalization, self-determination among those people, and empowerment as participants are empowered through their involvement in the arts (Nussbaum, 2011).

Recognizing the importance of the linkage between social work and the arts, and inspired by these three examplars, the Arts and Social Practice Conference was organized. Creating new opportunity structures for disadvantaged groups was seen as an avenue of social action with considerable strategic value for social workers operating at micro-, meso-, and macrolevels of practice.

The Design and Content of the Arts and Social Practice Conference

The inaugural Arts and Social Practice Conference, held at the University of Oklahoma on March 7, 2015, evolved as an effort to foster collaboration among professionals in the arts and practitioners in social service organizations. The event convened service providers, community leaders, artists, faculty, and students for a day of interactive discourse regarding the importance of arts engagement in communities. The conference presented social practice and the arts from clinical, cultural, and community perspectives, providing opportunities for participants to learn about the integration of the arts within community settings.

Conference Design

Conference conveners identified local professionals and service organizations doing creative work in diverse practice areas including aging, at-risk youth, homelessness, and mental illness. Through a needs assessment, the conference planning team identified 10 topical areas for the purpose of planning. The event was scheduled for a Saturday so that adequate campus facility space would be available at the university to support breakout sessions, forums, and large-group meetings.

It was recognized that although connections may be made at speaker sessions, as guests interact with the speakers, it is primarily through informal interactions among participants that such connections form. Indeed, one of the principal aims of the conference design was to bring into sustained interaction those who identify with the arts and those who identify with the helping professions. Relationship formation among group members who may not typically interact with one another served as a principal guidepost in conference design.

Conference Content

The conference began with a keynote address from the leader of a local arts organization who holds a graduate degree in social work. His speech, "Falling in Among Artists ... A Tale of Social Work," set the stage for the day's events. Morning breakout sessions included research on arts and neuroscience, presented by an academic researcher in social work; a joint presentation from Bring Back the Music and Elemental Hip Hop; two programs offering after-school programming for at-risk youth through music education; and a presentation from the Oklahoma Arts Council, providing guests with information on how the state organization assists local arts organizations to advance access to the arts.

During the second breakout session, representatives from the Cavett Kids Foundation offered content capturing the benefits of arts engagement for children who have life-threatening illnesses. The leader of Inclusion in Art demonstrated the importance of arts and inclusion, highlighting content on racial diversity in particular. The Homeless Alliance's Fresh stART program presented the value of arts access, and artistic development opportunities, for people who are homeless.

In the third session, the faculty of the University Writing Center under-scored how the arts can be useful in reaching people who experience trauma. Their presentation, titled "Survivors in Motion," illustrated the integration of the arts and mental health care through a digital storytelling workshop for survivors of recent Oklahoma tornadoes. Digital storytelling illustrated how the arts and mental health care can blend to reach those who experience trauma from natural disasters. A faculty member from the University's College of Architecture illustrated how arts engagement of seniors can facil-itate successful aging in community settings.

Evaluation of the Arts and Social Practice Conference

Evaluation included a triangulated approach involving the use of standar-dized continuing education evaluation forms, participant observation, and exit surveys. For the purposes of evaluation, the conveners collected data through 100 standardized evaluation forms from conference participants, narratives from 14 participant observers (who spent the day observing the conference workshops, forums, and events), and via 32 exit surveys. Themes that emerged regarding the tone of the event included diversity, engagement, enthusiasm, interest and curiosity, and motivation. Comments regarding diversity included 15 positive remarks addressing the demographic represen-tation, variety of speakers, and topics represented at the conference.

Narratives from participant observers, qualitative observations from stan-dardized speaker evaluations, and exit survey comments indicated that desired connections among participants did occur during the event. Overall, responses were overwhelmingly positive. As one participant noted, "The arts community and social organizations often think of themselves as separate entities. This was a chance to begin a dialogue about how the two go hand in hand." This statement reflected a typical response from participants.

The theme of successful integration of the arts with social practice was clearly illustrated within the qualitative data. Forty-six comments from exit surveys and participant observer narratives shared this theme. A sample exit survey comment was, "I was able to make connections as an upcoming social worker, and the various art events and how the two interact." Another important theme of the content analysis involved the intent of participants to apply information from the conference in practice settings. This sought-after outcome was significant, because a desired outcome of the conference was to foster integration of the arts into social service organizations. Nineteen comments were reflective of this theme.

The primary objective of the conference was to bring together profes-sionals from the arts community, social service organizations, and academia in order to begin a dialogue among diverse professionals who seek the integration of the arts, arts activism, and practice in the helping professions. Networking across disciplines was conceptualized as vital to this development and was a strong theme emerging from the qualitative data. One hundred sixteen comments focused on the overall theme of "interaction." A participant observer noted, "It seemed people were consistently making connections, meeting new people, and learning very valuable information."

Implications

Perhaps the most traditional approach to continuing education is to offer content on the state of practice in which social workers acquire the attitudes, skills, and competencies to engage within existing models. Such competence-based professional development can assist practicing social workers in becoming more familiar with present practice within social work so they can fill in the gaps in their professional portfolios.

Alternatively, continuing education in social work can anticipate new fields and domains of practice and offer innovations that can expand social workers' professional horizons. By offering learning experiences concerning emergent domains, continuing education can enable the profession to anticipate its own evolution into novel areas of practice (Huston, 2007; Scharmer, 2009). Over the history of social work, the profession has grown proactively by adapting its core model of helping to emerging areas of social need, with new solutions and social arrangements steering the helping process.

For us, the synergy of the arts and social practice represents such an emerging arena for social work practice in which the arts can become a vehicle for advancing human development, addressing social marginalization, and taking action to address persistent social inequity within society. Such synergy has the potential to bring social workers into collaboration with artists, community arts leaders, and other human service professionals committed to social change through the arts.

As we believe the Arts and Social Practice Conference may have illustrated, populations experiencing marginalization can gain benefits from the arts that they may be unable to experience through traditional social services. Continuing education, as a way of addressing such emergent opportunities, can create interactions among social workers and other professionals, activists, and cultural organizations that can stimulate new ways of engaging in the provision of assistance to those in need. Thus, perhaps the mission of continuing social work education can come to recognize its multiple functions—to diffuse good state-of-the-art practice knowledge, facilitate skill acquisition, and expand professional awareness about what may be novel ways of enacting helping.

References

Allen, P. (1995). *Art as a way of knowing.* Boston, MA: Shambhala.

Austen, H. (2010). *Artistry unleashed.* Toronto, Canada: University of Toronto Press.

Belfiore, E., & Bennett, O. (2008). *The social impact of the arts: An intellectual history.* New York, NY: Routledge.

Boeck, D., Moxley, D., & Wachter, H. (2011, January). *The infusion of the arts and humanities into a community needs assessment of aging: Rationale guiding the environmental design exhibit.* Proceedings of the 9th Hawaii International Conference on Arts and Humanities, Honolulu, HI.

Boylan, M. (2008). *The good, the true, and the beautiful: A quest for meaning.* London, UK: Continuum.

Brandt, D. (2008). Touching minds and hearts: Community arts as collaborative research. In G. J. Knowles & A. L. Cole (Eds.), *Handbook of arts in qualitative research: Perspectives, methodologies, examples and issues* (pp. 351–362). Thousand Oaks, CA: Sage.

Campana, A. (2011). Agents of possibility: Examining the intersections of art, education and activism in communities. *Studies in Art Education, 52,* 278–291.

Carey, J. (2006). *What good are the arts?* New York, NY: Oxford University Press.

Edwards, D. (2010a). *Artscience: Creativity in the post-Google generation.* Cambridge, MA: Harvard University Press.

Edwards, D. (2010b). *The lab: Creativity and culture.* Cambridge, MA: Harvard University Press.

Eisner, E. (1981). On the differences between scientific and artistic approaches to qualitative research. *Educational Researcher, 10*(4), 5–9. doi:10.3102/0013189X010004005

Eisner, E. W. (2004). *The arts and creation of mind.* New Haven, CT: Yale University Press.

Eisner, E. (2008). Art and knowledge. In G. J. Knowles & A. L. Cole (Eds.), *Handbook of arts in qualitative research: Perspectives, methodologies, examples and issues* (pp. 3–12). Thousand Oaks, CA: Sage.

Elmendorff, D. (2009). Minding our p's and q's: Addressing possibilities and precautions of community work through new questions. *Art Therapy: Journal of the American Art Therapy Association, 27*(1), 172–180.

Escobar, E. (1994). The heuristic power of art. In C. Becker (Ed.), *The subversive imagination: Artists, society and social responsibility* (pp. 35–54). New York, NY: Routledge.

Feen-Calligan, H., Washington, O., & Moxley, D. P. (2009). Homelessness among older African American women: Interpreting a serious social issue through the arts and education in community based participatory action research. *New Solutions, 19*(4), 423–448. doi:10.2190/NS.19.4.d

Harvey, J. (1996). *Embracing their memory: Loss and the social psychology of storytelling.* Needham Heights, MA: Allyn & Bacon.

Homeless Alliance. (2010). *Fresh stART.* Retrieved from http://homelessalliance.org/?page_id=1078

Huston, T. (2007). *Inside-Out: Stories and methods for generating collective will to create the future we want.* Cambridge, MA: Society for Organizational Learning.

Johnson, S. (2010). *Where good ideas come from: The natural history of innovation.* New York, NY: Riverhead Books.

Junge, M. B. (1999). Mourning memory and life itself: The AIDS quilt and the Vietnam Veterans memorial wall. *The Arts in Psychotherapy, 26,* 196–203.

Kaminsky, M. (1984). *The road from Hiroshima: A narrative poem.* New York, NY: Simon & Schuster.

Moxley, D. (2013). Incorporating art-making into the cultural practice of social work. *Journal of Ethnic and Cultural Diversity in Social Work*, *22*(3/4), 235–255. doi:10.1080/15313204.2013.843136

Moxley, D. (2014). Reflecting on the arts in social action: Possibilities for creative engagement in action learning. *Action Learning Action Research Journal*, *20*(1), 35–62.

Nussbaum, M. C. (2011). *Creating capabilities: The human development approach.* Cambridge, MA: Belknap Harvard.

Scharmer, C. O. (2009). *Theory U: Leading from the future as it emerges.* San Francisco, CA: Berrett-Kohler.

Sunstein, C. (2003). *Why societies need dissent.* Cambridge, MA: Harvard University Press.

Watkins, M., & Shulman, H. (2008). Liberation arts: Amnesia, counter memory, counter-memorial. In M. Watkins & H. Shulman (Eds.), *Toward psychologies of liberation* (pp. 232–265). New York, NY: Palgrave-MacMillan.

Zeisel, E. (2004). *On design: The magic language of things.* New York, NY: Overlook Duckworth.

Zinn, H. (2003). *Artists in time of war.* New York, NY: Seven Stories Press.

Creating a Continuing Education Pathway for Newly Arrived Immigrants and Refugee Communities

Aster S. Tecle, An Thi Ha, and Rosemarie Hunter

ABSTRACT

With the increase in the number of displaced peoples, the demand for skilled social workers from diverse backgrounds to serve them is critical. This article explores a continuing education program that prepares precollege individuals from newly arriving communities who will work as entry-level workers serving these immigrant and refugee communities. The article focuses on the development of a Case Management Certificate Program as a response to community-identified issues, then presents a discussion exploring the educational pathways and unique contributions of these individuals. The article calls for the profession to explore how continuing education pathways can bridge service gaps, contribute to the knowledge base of social work, and meet current labor market demands.

Introduction

At the end of 2014, the number of forcibly displaced individuals worldwide was 59.5 million (United Nations High Commissioner for Refugees [UNHCR], 2015), and there were 19.5 million individuals with refugee status worldwide at the beginning of 2013 (UNHCR, 2014). The exodus of people from their homelands and the rapidly increasing trend of regional and global forced migrations have raised the resettlement ceiling for the United States to 85,000 for 2016 and 100,000 in 2017 (Population, Refugees and Migration, 2016). The main contributors to forced migration vary, ranging from globalization to climate change, with armed conflicts and war ranking as the major contributing forces. By the end of 2014, top ranking source of refugees were Syria (currently 4.25 million Internally Displaced Peoples), Afghanistan (one of four refugees in the world), Somalia, Iraq, and South Sudan (UNHCR, 2014). Resettled communities thus come from different continents wherein the sociopolitical, economic, and military conditions forced them to migrate in search of a decent life and security. The condition of forcibly displaced peoples and migrants calls for urgent responses to a global crisis, not only as a humanitarian issue but also as a human rights issue.

Growing global inequality, social exclusion, and violence in the 21st century are challenging social work ideals of social justice (Finn, 2013; Finn and Jacobson, 2003). Forced migration results from historically oppressive local and global conditions that have long-term impacts. Those forced to migrate from their homelands are diverse and thus their demands more complex. In the resettlement processes, cultural diversity, socioeconomic differences, and migrants' political consciousness inform their demands and expectations from host societies (Waters, 1999). Although rarely recognized, migrants' backgrounds are often replete with diverse professions, skills and experiences that can contribute to host societies. Their professions range from physicians, engineers, nurses, and researchers to social workers, teachers, and public service providers. Too often their expertise remains invisible to host societies due to a lack of recognition of their professions by Western educational institutions and to requirements to upgrade their academic credits and accomplishments. In addition, there are stereotypes attached to refugees and immigrants from Latin America, Asia, Africa, and the Middle East (Perry and Mallozzi, 2011). As for the cultural aspect, people from the global south are already imagined as "lacking," backward, and traditional, which calls for resettled people to "catch up" with the modern world (Escobar, 1995; Said, 1979). Yet most refugees are well educated and highly credentialed before they come to the United States (Anderson, Purcell-Gates, Gagne, & Jang, 2009; Barton, Ivanic, Appleby, Hodge, & Tustin, 2007; Fingeret & Drennon, as cited in Smyth & Kum, 2010).

The opportunity to pursue basic literacy and higher education frequently motivates immigrants and refugees to resettle in a third country (Perry, 2010). However, similar to other adult learners, educational and employment barriers often block them from pursuing their goals (Kerwin, 2009). Hence, post-resettlement processes tend to force them to accept manufacturing or low-wage service sector jobs regardless of their previous experience and profession (Kenny, 2011). The U.S. Office of Refugee Resettlement's policy of promoting refugee self-sufficiency within a short time via employment has been questioned in terms of whether it is realistic and appropriate (Brick et al., 2010; International Rescue Committee, 2009; Perry, 2010; Presse & Thompson, 2007; Wright, 1981). Beyond existing job trainings and English Language Learning classes for employment purposes, educational opportunities that would have refined the expertise of the immigrants and refugees to meet local demands do not appear to be included in the policy vision. The "one-size-fits-all" approach has not worked well in meeting the variety of refugees and immigrants' demands (Kerwin, 2011; Perry, 2008). Policy recommendations suggest that, in addition to employment opportunities, education is the main focus and indicator of resettlement expected outcomes (Brick et al., 2010).

The unsettling 21st-century global reality requires that social work education develop innovative programs that will adequately prepare resettled refugees and immigrants to practice with diverse communities and in complex sociopolitical settings. Due to geographic, cultural, and socioeconomic divides, more often than not migrants are insufficiently exposed to other parts of the globe and therefore lack the skills of navigating resettlement systems and institutions. The social work profession thus has the responsibility to prepare resettled paraprofessionals. There is a need for future generations of American social workers to be able to acknowledge migrants' cultures and knowledge as equally legitimate as their own and to design programs that will prepare members of resettled communities to engage in foundational social service providing professions.

The Case Management Certificate Program (CMCP) at the University of Utah is one such attempt in social work. CMCP provides the knowledge and skills required to provide services to the next wave of immigrants and refugees in Salt Lake City, the knowledge gained from this program is making a new contribution to social work education at the local university. Developed as a response to the initiatives and demands of resettled communities, the CMCP is located in one of the city's most diverse and lower socioeconomic neighborhoods. Capacity-building and empowerment frameworks, whereby resettled communities take charge of their own affairs, are central to the program. This article explores the development and teaching-learning process of a 9-month continuing education certificate offering a conceptualized paraprofessional, precollege case management program designed for newly arriving migrants. The aim is not only to build bridges between resettled communities and service providing institutions but also for host societies to reframe their perceptions about locally globally resettled communities from "social welfare dependents" to paraprofessional colleagues who will contribute to and serve their communities and hence the host society.

The first section of this article focuses on theoretical frameworks, followed by the context and the nature of the CMCP. The program is administered by the University of Utah, College of Social Work, Professional and Community Education Program. The final sections conclude the article with a discussion on educational pathways.

The Theoretical Frameworks of the CMCP

The CMCP is a continuing education certificate program and pathway grounded in the theories and foundations of continuing education, adult learning theory, and action learning.

Continuing Education

Continuing education is defined by Halton, Powell, and Scanlon (2014) as lifelong learning or "an ongoing process of education and development that continues throughout the professional's career" (p. 1). The rapid changes of social phenomena, professional knowledge, and technological innovation require social workers to adapt in order to be prepared for practice. The realities have led to the need for social workers' commitments to continuing professional education in order to critically reflect on and continuously update themselves with respect to emerging knowledge and innovations (Congress, 2012; Halton et al., 2014; Lary & Duffey, 2000; National Association of Social Workers [NASW], 2003).

In the United States, continuing education is a requirement for social workers' licensure renewal in all 50 states (NASW, 2011; Quinn & Straussner, 2010). To guide social workers and stakeholders, the NASW developed the standards for continuing education (NASW, 2003) and the guidelines for continuing education program approval (NASW, 2011). Continuing professional education can be formal (i.e., courses, workshops, practice-oriented seminars) or informal (i.e., supervision, readings, publications, reflection and peer support) (Congress, 2012; Halton et al., 2014; NASW, 2003).

The effectiveness of continuing education programs has been demonstrated through empirical studies. Quinn and Straussner (2010) found that a continuing education program on substance abuse enhanced social workers' competencies in working with this population and assisted in providing a more ethical provision of services. A workshop on evidence-based practice also resulted in changes in participants' views, knowledge, and self-reported behavior regarding the evidence-based practice process (Parrish & Rubin, 2011). Similarly, according to Halton et al. (2014), the vast majority of survey participants who were International Association of Schools of Social Work members indicated that attending continuing professional courses such as in-service training and professional courses had been either "helpful" or "very helpful" in their work, with "other professional courses" earning the highest rating (98%), followed by higher education (91%) and in-service training (86%). In brief, continuing education is perceived as an essential way for social workers to develop and improve their professional and employment performance.

Continuing education also acknowledges the employees' commitments and responsibilities for advancing and renewing knowledge, skills, belief, and values in social work. This continuing education philosophy reinforces the CMCP's mission of providing those who engage in case management and community practice with knowledge, skills, and values relevant to their work and needed to provide quality service.

Andragogy—An Adult Learning Theory

The term *andragogy* is well known as Malcolm Knowles's theory of adult learning. Andragogy (often contrasted to pedagogy, which is considered the "art and science of teaching children") is described as "the art and science of helping adults learn" (Knowles, Holton, & Swanson, 1998, p. 61). Knowles's theory offered six assumptions about the characteristics of adult learners different from youth learners: (a) adults consider the value and the necessity of learning something before learning new things, (b) adults acknowledge their responsibilities for their own decisions, (c) adults bring more and different experience than youth to the classroom, (d) adults have motivation to learn things important to them and to apply what they learn in a real-life situation, (e) adults are life centered or problem centered in their learning orientations, and (f) adults are motivated more by internal pressures than external factors.

Knowles also suggested four principles to apply in adult learning (Smith, 2010): (a) engaging adults in the planning and evaluation of the courses, (b) the significance of experiential learning, (c) the immediate relevance of learning subjects to learners' lives, and (d) applying problem-centered approaches instead of content-oriented approaches. In other words, adult learning included an emphasis on independence, self-direction, experience, flexibility, and feedback. Understanding these characteristics (and applying them to designing continuing education programs) will likely promote a program's appropriateness and effectiveness.

Jack Mezirow is another well-known name in the adult learning arena. Mezirow (1985) emphasized the importance of including dialogue, self-directed learning, and learners' needs and interests. His work raises the significance of interaction, reflection, and continued need assessments in order to discover the learners' real interests, which is central to designing a learning process that will strengthen the learner's ability to "become increasingly autonomous and responsible" (p. 142). Mezirow argued that adult learning is not just a process of updating personal knowledge. Rather, it facilitates social action, which encourages learners to "become aware of the cultural contradictions which oppress them, research their own problems, build confidence, examine action alternatives, identify resources, anticipate consequences, foster participation and leadership and assess relevant experience" (p. 149).

Like Knowles and Mezirow, Marienau and Reed (2008) paid attention to learners' assumptions, beliefs, and commitment, as well as the value of experiential learning, reflection on experience, a problem-orientation, and social relationships. Geron, Andrews, and Hun (2005), reflecting a similar view to Knowles with regard to adult learners' characteristics, suggested that equipping them with knowledge and research findings is not adequate. Strengthening them with practical skills, providing them with opportunities to reflect and explore their beliefs and values, and empowering them in the process are crucial goals of adult learning.

By gaining insights about adult learning theories, we acknowledged the CMCP participants as adult learners, with their own knowledge, experience, and backgrounds.

Action Learning

Action learning is grounded in the ideology of learning by doing; learning from experience; or learning by solving problems through teamwork, project focus, and reflection (Cho & Egan, 2009; Marsick & O'Neil, 1999; O'Neil & Marsick, 2014; Pedler, 2011; Revans, 1982, 2011). In particular, Revans (1982) defined action learning as a means of "development, intellectual, emotional or physical, that requires its subjects, through responsible involvement in some real, complex and stressful problem, to achieve intended change to improve their observable behavior henceforth in the problem field" (pp. 626–627). As pointed out by Pedler, "there is no learning without action and no sober and deliberate action without learning" (as cited in Marsick & O'Neil, 1999, pp. xxii–xxiii). Although learning provides individuals with programmed knowledge, action (case studies, live projects, simulation exercises, or adventure activities) produces opportunities to question and reflect such programmed knowledge through real situations and experiences. In addition, by participating in a small group for action, participants learn from and reflect with their peers (Cho & Egan, 2009; Revans, 2011).

As opposed to traditional lecture-oriented programs, action learning employs adult education theories (Cho & Egan, 2009). Proponents of this approach believe that people learn most effectively through working on real problems existing in their own employment setting (Cho & Egan, 2009; O'Neil & Marsick, 2014; Revans, 2011) and reflecting critically with peers, colleagues, or instructors. Based on these pedagogical notions, training programs for adults, such as the Utah School of Social Work's CMCP, encourage the active participation of enrollees while instructors play a role as facilitators, supporting an action-learning environment.

Emerging Leaders Project

The Community Context

The *Emerging Leaders Project*, the development phase of the CMCP, began in 2012 as a response to requests by the Utah State Office of Refugee Services, resettlement agencies, and social service agencies to support the integration of newly arriving communities of immigrants and refugees. Salt Lake City has a rich history of serving as a gateway community for new arriving populations from all over the world, hosting approximately 50,000 refugees, with more than 1,000 new arrivals each year. In 2014, for example, the City received 1,286 refugees (Utah Department of Health, 2014). The community focus for the Emerging Leaders Project included the City's most diverse and rapidly growing neighborhoods. An area report conducted by

University Neighborhood Partners (2012) identified that almost 36% of the City's total population lives in the River District (west side)—66,701 people out of the City's total population of 186,440. The report also noted that the population in this area grew by 10.7%, compared to an overall 2.6% growth for Salt Lake City. Additional growth was seen in the share of River District residents who are identified as "minority," moving from 52% in 2000 to more than 62% in 2010. The River District is home to a large Latino/a population, with 46% of the population identifying as Hispanic, to 83% of the City's Pacific Islanders, and 60.8% of the City's Black population (UNP Report, 2012).

Ethnic Community-Based Organizations

In response to the large number (and rich diversity) of newly arriving individuals, a consortium of social service agencies, resettlement organizations, and grassroots leaders collaborated to develop an initiative to support the development of Ethnic Community-Based Organizations – such as the Bhutanese Community Association, Latino Behavioral Health, Sudanese Association of Utah. The goals of these community-based organizations are to provide support to arriving individuals and to act as an information, referral, and crisis response network, connecting new arriving populations to existing resources and systems (Hunter & Mileski, 2013). Many social service organizations also were interested in members of these ECBOs serving as "bridge workers," having the cultural knowledge and linguistic skills needed to support new arrivals in navigating local systems in order to access services, employment, and education. We learned that individuals organizing in their own ethnic communities also are employed in entry-level positions (as case managers, youth and family liaisons, employment counselors) in schools, at resettlement agencies, and with social service providers. Because they are already recognized members in their own communities, such individuals have the potential of understanding the unique needs and strengths of their own communities and the cultural issues present (Hunter, Mai, Hollister, & Jankey, 2011). In this way, they occupy a shared status across both the host and ethnic communities.

Nevertheless, although community-based leaders come with existing skills, they also often understandably have a novice understanding of Western systems and often lack professional credentials that are recognized in the United States. The Emerging Leaders Project included a yearlong process utilizing a participatory action research framework to better understand the educational strengths and needs of these individuals that would assist them with acquiring entry-level positions in social service agencies, thereby creating a new pathway to enter the social work profession. One of the outcomes of the Emerging Leaders Project was the development of the CMCP (Hunter & Mileski, 2013).

The Curriculum

Located in a community-based setting, the CMCP includes the following four courses: Introduction to Social Work for Case Managers, Introduction to Interpersonal Communication & Documentation, Introduction to Casework, and Introduction to Community Practice and Advocacy. Each course, herein Phase 1, is taught by social work faculty in a weekly 3-hour block and meets for 8 weeks, creating a 9-month program. Interested participants complete an application process including the University's Continuing Education application form, a personal statement, and a letter of recommendation. (This project was deemed exempt from needing human subjects approval by the University of Utah's Institutional Review Board.)

The four social work courses that compose the CMCP were developed as part of the Emerging Leaders Project. Phase 2 of the project includes a participatory action research process—engaging with stakeholders from social service agencies, resettlement organizations, and members of the ECBOs—to identify agency and community needs and priorities. The four social work courses were developed within capacity building and empowerment frameworks, striving to be inclusive of all voices. The curriculum follows the tenants of adult learning theory and emphasizes applied learning for social change. Furthermore, social change agents are viewed from a wide scope of cultural perspectives, building on multiple ways of knowing and the rich history and knowledge of the students. Social work values are introduced in the first course and continue as a foundational learning objective in all courses. Learning from a generalist perspective, upon completion of CMCP students are able to understand and apply basic social work theory and skills; communicate effectively with individuals, families, and communities; understand and apply common case management principles, processes, and responsibilities in a multicultural context; and act as systemic change agents in ways that empower individuals, families, and groups.

The CMCP makes use of an applied curriculum in which participants are actively engaged in their communities. In this way, the CMCP may serve as a catalyst for social change in the communities where the students live. A case example would be CMCP's Introduction to Community Practice and Advocacy course project conducted with the Bhutanese community and a diverse group of CMCP students. Traditionally, there are expectations from school systems in the United States such as (a) teachers and parents work together, and (b) parents are expected to participate in their child's education, set expectations, and attend parent–teacher conferences. This project, therefore, explored families' frustrations with local schools that haven't been able to bridge the school–home, teacher–student, and parent–school gaps. According to the Bhutanese participants in the project, these parents expressed the felt need for support systems to better understand the school system. They further identified issues related to communication barriers, lack of strict rules and regulations for students who miss classes, use of mobile phones in the classroom, and dressing codes. Similarly, there was frustration with the age-based assignment to grade schools for children who have spent most of their childhood with little (if any) formal education, and the need to teach subject content and English language together in order to assist them with understanding concepts in a particular subject. Parents also shared the importance of the recognition of their cultures as being critical to the learning process of their children, and with strengthening parent–child communication. Finally, these parents identified very demanding jobs as barriers to engaging in their children's lives. Project participants summarized some of the learning, presented next.

> Day by day children are out of control of their parents and the culture, which has impacted their further education. They are motivated to making money and getting married at early ages. Once the family has started growing, the financial burden comes to a head, so they cannot think of further education. (CMCP Team 6, 2014)

Early marriage also was identified as contributing to girls' lack of retention in school. The Plan of Action the team designed included the following:

> Education is a very crucial part of communal growth and development. We would like to submit these issues to our community leaders to research more on these issues and act accordingly; schedule a date convenient to all high school children and discuss this issue one more time for education is a broad system and the voice of a couple of students does not bring any changes. The time frame assigned to do this is three months.

These are a few examples of the critical issues that CMCP students raise and advocate for as agents of social change in their communities. These students are working as "bridge builders," case managers, interpreters, and organizers within their respective communities, addressing the need to bring people together, build broad based power, trust and diversified leadership in their communities, and assist in navigating systems (Pyles, 2014; Shaw, 2014).

The Student Body as Social Change Agents

Now in its 3rd year (2014–2016), the student body of the CMCP is very diverse and continues to be involved in a wide variety of systems work. Enrollment has been increasing (from 28 students in the first cohort to 36 students in the third cohort), despite the fact that a few students from the second and third cohorts dropped out due to family or work obligations and the lack of time to come to class straight from work. The student body comprises refugees and immigrants from developing countries (global south) and Eastern Europe. The demographics of the three cohorts is 34 female students and 48 male students (82 total) from 21 countries located in the following continents (and regions): Africa (36), the Middle East (eight), Asia (22, includes SW Asia and South Central: two from Iran and one from Afghanistan, respectively), Latin America (13), Eastern Europe (one), and the United States (two). On average, students' age ranged from 12 students who were younger than 30 (14.6%), 36 students 30–39 years old (43.9%), 21 students 40 to 49 years old (25.7%), and 13 students who were 50 years of age or older (15.8%).

Early data from program evaluations and a more detailed impact study (currently in progress) indicate that the CMCP serves as both an employment and social work education pathway for individuals of immigrant and refugee background. In a program evaluation meeting with representatives of the Utah Office of Refugee Services, participants reported that graduates are increasingly securing entry-level positions. In addition, a focus group with graduates from the first and second cohorts shared examples of graduates pursuing higher education at the associate's and BSW levels. There is also early evidence of an increase in the organizational capacity of ECBOs. For example, several graduates of the first and second cohorts continue to partner and share resources to host community events and workshops. In one case, Bhutanese graduates of the first cohort are partnering with Latino graduates on training community members in the National Alliance on Mental Illness Family-to-Family support model (J. Gomez-Aries, personal communication, November 24, 2015).

Discussion

Emerging Continuing Education Pathways

Newly arriving communities come from diverse backgrounds, yet their heterogeneity frequently has been considered a barrier to moving forward rather than a cultural wealth to harness. The most difficult hurdle they face is deprofessionalization, loss of their profession, or lack of opportunity to access educational institutions due to discriminatory practices and rigid systemic barriers (Smyth & Kum, 2010). Deprofessionalization and disqualification of members of newly arriving communities may in turn call for investments in education but may not reflect their cultural capital. Hence, there is a need for the social work profession to support members of newly arriving communities reenter their profession.

As noted, there is a need for the social work profession to design paraprofessional continuing education, community-based, and action-oriented programs to engage these communities. The aim is to strengthen and systematize practice with newly arriving communities and introduce critical thinking to their practical approaches. Such a framework to continuing education demands that the social work profession expand its vision and mission statement to employ a community-based, participatory, and empowering framework, building on a broad base of community knowledge, skill, and wisdom. Such a paraprofessional social work continuing education program for newly arrived immigrants and refugees creates an educational pathway to higher education in social work that will strengthen the profession. The program will also contribute to promoting social work practice with diverse communities, as well as promoting an expansion of social change agents in the profession and public institutions.

A wide range of public institutions and nongovernmental agencies are involved in supporting newly arriving communities in the areas of health, education, housing, transportation, and employment. Having social work paraprofessionals working with these agencies addresses current language, cultural, and systemic issues that are costly to both service providers and clients served.

Limitations

The CMCP developed as a response to one city's desire to provide improved services to new arriving communities of immigrants and refugees. At the same time, the Participatory Action Research framework applied in this project centered the *voices* of those most affected by their new circumstances. The resulting continuing education certificate program was specifically designed for this Salt Lake City setting, and consequently there is no certainty about how this program might be applied with other urban or rural communities or with other newly arrived populations.

An additional limitation of the study is the lack of existing research on the precollege pathway in the arena of social work continuing education. Although there are an abundance of certificate programs in social work, there is a lack of literature on the intentional use of precollege programs to support a new pathway and thus the extension of the role social work continuing education. Furthermore, the authors acknowledge that the discussion of paraprofessional levels of social work education is complex and political. Indeed, we question whether the term "paraprofessional" is even appropriate.

Similarly, because of the newness of this project, the findings are preliminary. There must be longitudinal investigation of the impact to provide evidence of effectiveness. Equally important would be to measure (a) how the program contributes to systems change and (b) the integration of new knowledge into social service delivery programs serving newly resettled communities. We look to the graduates of the first two cohorts, and the stakeholder groups engaged in this project, to support us in learning more about how to best define this work and its place in social work education.

Conclusion

As current trends of global migration illustrate, the number of refugees and immigrants seeking to come to America will rise. Some likely will be highly educated professionals, whereas others will have only basic skills and literacy. Consequently, there is a need for higher education institutions both to recognize their expertise and to equip them with skills that will transform their quality of life. The CMCP calls for the expansion of social work continuing education to better serve resettled communities, which in turn will contribute to the hosting society. Exploring their knowledge and expertise, based on community-driven approaches, is key to bridging the gaps between service providers and resettled communities as well as meeting emerging labor market demands. As CMCP indicates, the conceptualization of the program, diversity of the student body, and their communities' contributions to the design of the program have enriched this particular certificate program beyond expectations. Graduates now are working with service providing agencies as "bridge builders," thus facilitating resettlement processes.

Rather than "starting from scratch," a program design should seek to create a vehicle for the validation of resettled communities' expertise and life experience while assisting members to move forward with their credentials. Equally important is the current need within the social work profession to recruit a diverse workforce, explore how emerging cross-cultural expertise can inform social work pedagogy, and address how new content rich in appreciation for diversity can be integrated into the curriculum.

References

Anderson, J., Purcell-Gates, V., Gagne, M., & Jang, K. (2009). *Implementing an intergenerational literacy program with authentic literacy instruction: Challenges, responses, and results.* Vancouver, Canada: University of British Columbia.

Barton, D., Ivanic, R., Appleby, Y., Hodge, R., & Tustin, K. (2007). *Literacy, lives and learning.* London, UK: Routledge.

Brick, K., Krill, A., Cushing-Savvi, A., Scanlon, M. M., Elshafie, S., & Stone, M. (2010). *Refugee Resettlement in the United States: An examination of challenges and proposed solutions.* New York, NY: Columbia University School of International and Public Affairs.

Case Management Certificate Program. (2014, Spring). College of Social Work. Students' Social Change Effort Project, Team 6 (Unpublished course project). Salt Lake City: College of Social Work, University of Utah.

Cho, Y., & Egan, T. M. (2009). Action learning research: A systematic review and conceptual framework. *Human Resource Development Review, 8*(4), 431–462.

Congress, E. P. (2012). Continuing education: Lifelong learning for social work practitioners and educators. *Journal of Social Work Education, 48*(3), 397–401. doi:10.517/SJSWE.2012.201200085

Escobar, A. (1995). *Encountering development: The making and unmaking of the third world.* Princeton, NJ: Princeton University Press.

Finn, J. and Jacobson, M. (2003). Just Practice: Steps Towards A New Social Work Paradigm. *Journal of Social Work Education, 39*(1).

Finn, J. and Jacobson, M. (2013). Social Justice. In T. Mizrahi and L. Davis (Eds.), *Encyclopedia of Social Work*, Oxford University Press. DOI: 10.1093/acrefore/9780199975839.013.364.

Finn, J. L., & Jacobson, M. (2008). *Just practice: A social justice approach to social work.* Peosta, IA: Eddie Bowers.

Geron, S. M., Andrews, C., & Hun, K. (2005). Infusing aging skills into the social work practice community: A new look at strategies for continuing professional education. *Families in Society: The Journal of Contemporary Social Services, 86*(3), 431–440. doi:10.1606/1044-3894.3442

Halton, C., Powell, F., & Scanlon, M. (2014). *Continuing professional development in social work.* Bristol, UK: Policy Press.

Hunter, R., Mai, T., Hollister, L., & Jankey, O. (2011). A university-community partnership model for capacity-building and collective learning with individuals of immigrant and refugee experience: The example of the Hartland partnership center. *Journal of Global Social Work Practice, 4*(1). Retrieved from http://www.globalsocialwork.org/vol4no1/Hunter.html

Hunter, R., & Mileski, K. (2013). Emerging leaders project: Connecting university resources to community-based organizations supporting refugee resettlement. *Advances in Social Work, 14*(2), 613–628.

International Rescue Committee. (2009). *World Refugee Day, 2009.* Retrieved from http://www.rescue.org/world-refugee-day-2009

Kenny, P. (2011). A mixed blessing: Karen resettlement to the United States. *Journal of Refugee Studies, 24*, 217–238. doi:10.1093/jrs/fer009

Kerwin, D. (2009). Rights, the common good, and sovereignty in service of the human person. In D. Kerwin & J. M. Gerschutz (Eds.), *And you welcomed me: Migration and catholic social teaching* (pp. 93–121). Lanham, MD: Lexington Books.

Kerwin, D. (2011). *The faltering US refugee protection system: Legal and policy responses to refugees, asylum seekers, and others in need of protection.* New York, NY: Migration Policy Institute.

Knowles, M. S., Holton, III, E. F., & Swanson, R. A. (1998). *The adult learner: The definitive classic in adult education and human resource development.* Houston, TX: Gulf Publishing Co.

Lary, C. J., & Duffey, S. (2000). *Philosophical foundations: A primer for adult continuing education.* Washington, DC: Educational Resources Information Center.

Marienau, C., & Reed, S. C. (2008). Educator as designer: Balancing multiple teaching perspectives in the design of community based learning for adults. *New Directions for Adult and Continuing Education, 18*, 60–74.

Marsick, V. J., & O'Neil, J. (1999). The many faces of action learning. *Management Learning, 30*(2), 159–176. doi:10.1177/1350507699302004

Mezirow, J. (1985). Concept and action in adult education. *Adult Education Quarterly, 35*(3), 142–151. doi:10.1177/0001848185035003003

National Association of Social Workers. (2003). *NASW standards for continuing professional education.* Washington, DC: Author.

National Association of Social Workers. (2011). *Continuing education approval program guidelines.* Washington, DC: Author.

O'Neil, J., & Marsick, V. J. (2014). Action learning coaching. *Advances in Developing Human Resources, 16*(2), 202–221. doi:10.1177/1523422313520202

Parrish, D. E., & Rubin, A. (2011). An effective model for continuing education training in evidence-based practice. *Research on Social Work Practice, 21*(1), 77–87. doi:10.1177/1049731509359187

Pedler, M. (2011). *Action learning in practice.* Brookfield, VT: Gower.

Perry, K. H. (2008). From storytelling to writing: Transforming literacy practices among Sudanese refugees. *Journal of Literacy Research, 40*(4), 317–358. doi:10.1080/10862960802502196

Perry, K. H. (2010). *Adult literacy and ESL provision in Lexington*. Lexington, KY: Collaborative Center on Literacy Development.

Perry, K. H., & Mallozzi, C. (2011). 'Are you able to learn?' Power and access to higher education for African refugees in the U.S.. *Power and Education, 3*(3), 249–262. doi:10.2304/power.2011.3.3.249

Population, Refugees and Migration. (2016). Myths and facts on refugees, migration, and humanitarian assistance. Retrieved from http://www.state.gov/j/prm/releases/factsheets/2016/255967.htm

Presse, D., & Thompson, J. (2007). The resettlement challenge: Integration of refugees from protracted refugee situations. *Refuge, 24*(2), 94–99.

Pyles, L. (2014). *Progressive community organizing*. New York, NY: Routledge.

Quinn, G., & Straussner, S. L. A. (2010). Licensure and continuing education requirements for substance abuse training in social work. *Journal of Social Work Practice in the Addictions, 10*, 433–437. doi:10.1080/1533256X.2010.521084

Revans, R. W. (1982). *The origins and growth of action learning*. London, UK: Chartwell-Bratt.

Revans, R. (2011). *ABC of action learning*. Brookfield, VT: Gower.

Said, E. (1979). *Orientalism*. New York, NY: Vintage Books.

Shaw, S. (2014). Bridge builders: A qualitative study exploring the experiences of former refugees working as case workers in the United States. *Journal of Social Service Research, 40*, 284–296. doi:10.1080/01488376.2014.901276

Smith, M. K. (2010). *'Andragogy,' the encyclopaedia of informal education*. Retrieved from http://infed.org/mobi/andragogy-what-is-it-and-does-it-help-thinking-about-adult-learning/

Smyth, G., & Kum, H. (2010). 'When they don't use it, they will lose it': Professionals, deprofessionalization, and reprofessionalization: The case of refugee teachers in Scotland. *Journal of Refugee Studies, 23*(4), 503–522. doi:10.1093/jrs/feq041

United Nations High Commissioner for Refugees. (2014). *Global trend: Forced displacement in 2014*. New York, NY: UN Press.

United Nations High Commissioner for Refugees. (2015). *Annual report 2015*. New York, NY: UN Press.

University Neighborhood Partners. (2012). *Annual report 2012*. Retrieved from http://partners.utah.edu/wp-content/uploads/UNP-Report-Spring-2012.pdf

Utah Department of Health. (2014). *Utah Bureau of Epidemiology Refugee Health Program*. Retrieved from http://health.utah.gov/epi/healthypeople/refugee/datastatistics/2014/age.pdf

Waters, M. C. (1999). *Black identities: West Indian immigrant dreams and American realities*. Cambridge, MA: Harvard University Press.

Wright, R. G. (1981). Voluntary agencies and the resettlement of refugees. *International Migration Review, 15*(1/2), 157–174. doi:10.2307/2545334

Index

Printed and bound by CPI Group (UK) Ltd, Croydon, CR0 4YY

01/11/2024

01782600-0006